Contents

Preface

Fast Facts for the Pediatric Nurse: An Orientation Guide in a Nutshell is designed for nurses who are beginning to work in the rewarding, yet sometimes challenging, field of pediatrics. The book can be a great asset to the novice nurse who is orienting to the unit, or even to the student nurse who is beginning a clinical rotation in the specialized area of pediatric nursing. This book was written by real nurses who presently care for, and teach the care of, children in times of health as well as illness.

Since children are not little adults, the nursing care of children is much different than medical–surgical nursing care of adults. A toddler who does not understand the need for care may kick, scream, and even bite in an effort to get away from the nurse. Learning how to assist with painful procedures that result in tears for the child and parents can be difficult and emotionally taxing for everyone involved. After all, caring for a crying child is intimidating and can upset even the seasoned nurse. This book presents suggestions on how to communicate and work with children using age-appropriate techniques. The authors share time-tested and proven tips to assist the new nurse in transition to becoming a pediatric nurse.

This book is formatted to allow for quick access to information. The frequently used terminology that is referenced in the index includes diseases and illnesses in childhood. In addition, the book is filled with *must-know* information on disease processes and clinical advice that come from years of experience.

Each chapter begins with a brief introduction and key chapter objectives. The content is arranged according to body systems and contains details of the most common illnesses within each system. The list of diagnoses includes descriptions, manifestations, diagnostic criteria, and interventions, each clearly listed and easy to understand. The Fast Facts in a Nutshell boxes are highlighted and provide focused, key clinical tips within each chapter. The information in this book is compiled from basic pediatric knowledge, and the sources are believed to be reliable and reflective of the most current evidence-based practice.

To be successful in pediatric nursing, the nurse must possess a fondness for children and a caring attitude. Yes, attitude is everything! No one expects the nurse to know everything, as nurses are human. Even when the nurse is falling to pieces on the inside, it's important to keep the parents calm, for calmness is catching. Rely on a preceptor or mentor that you trust, and always, always ask questions. Before long, you, the novice nurse, will become a mentor to another pediatric-minded nurse!

Diana Rupert
Kathleen Young

Fast Facts for the NEW NURSE PRACTITIONER: *What You Really Need to Know in a Nutshell*, Aktan

Fast Facts for the ER NURSE: *Emergency Room Orientation in a Nutshell, 2e,* Buettner

Fast Facts for the MEDICAL–SURGICAL NURSE: *Clinical Orientation in a Nutshell,* Ciocco

Fast Facts for the ANTEPARTUM AND POSTPARTUM NURSE: *A Nursing Orientation and Care Guide in a Nutshell,* Davidson

Fast Facts for the NEONATAL NURSE: *A Nursing Orientation and Care Guide in a Nutshell,* Davidson

Fast Facts About PRESSURE ULCER CARE FOR NURSES: *How to Prevent, Detect, and Resolve Them in a Nutshell,* Dziedzic

Fast Facts for the GERONTOLOGY NURSE: *A Nursing Care Guide in a Nutshell,* Eliopoulos

Fast Facts for the CLINICAL NURSE MANAGER: *Managing a Changing Workplace in a Nutshell,* Fry

Fast Facts for EVIDENCE-BASED PRACTICE: *Implementing EBP in a Nutshell,* Godshall

Fast Facts About NURSING AND THE LAW: *Law for Nurses in a Nutshell,* Grant, Ballard

Fast Facts for the L&D NURSE: *Labor & Delivery Orientation in a Nutshell,* Groll

Fast Facts for the RADIOLOGY NURSE: *An Orientation and Nursing Care Guide in a Nutshell,* Grossman

Fast Facts on ADOLESCENT HEALTH FOR NURSING AND HEALTH PROFESSIONALS: *A Care Guide in a Nutshell,* Herrman

Fast Facts for the FAITH COMMUNITY NURSE: *Implementing FCN/Parish Nursing in a Nutshell,* Hickman

Fast Facts for the CARDIAC SURGERY NURSE: *Everything You Need to Know in a Nutshell,* Hodge

Fast Facts for the CLINICAL NURSING INSTRUCTOR: *Clinical Teaching in a Nutshell, 2e,* Kan, Stabler-Haas

Fast Facts for the WOUND CARE NURSE: *Practical Wound Management in a Nutshell,* Kifer

Fast Facts About EKGs FOR NURSES: *The Rules of Identifying EKGs in a Nutshell,* Landrum

Fast Facts for the CRITICAL CARE NURSE: *Critical Care Nursing in a Nutshell,* Landrum

Fast Facts for the TRAVEL NURSE: *Travel Nursing in a Nutshell,* Landrum

Fast Facts for the SCHOOL NURSE: *School Nursing in a Nutshell,* Loschiavo

Fast Facts About CURRICULUM DEVELOPMENT IN NURSING: *How to Develop & Evaluate Educational Programs in a Nutshell,* McCoy, Anema

Fast Facts for DEMENTIA CARE: *What Nurses Need to Know in a Nutshell,* Miller

Fast Facts for HEALTH PROMOTION IN NURSING: *Promoting Wellness in a Nutshell,* Miller

Fast Facts for STROKE CARE NURSING: *An Expert Guide in a Nutshell,* Morrison

Fast Facts for the MEDICAL OFFICE NURSE: *What You Really Need to Know in a Nutshell,* Richmeier

Fast Facts for the PEDIATRIC NURSE: *An Orientation Guide in a Nutshell,* Rupert, Young

Fast Facts About the GYNECOLOGICAL EXAM FOR NURSE PRACTITIONERS: *Conducting the GYN Exam in a Nutshell*, Secor, Fantasia

Fast Facts for the STUDENT NURSE: *Nursing Student Success in a Nutshell*, Stabler-Haas

Fast Facts for CAREER SUCCESS IN NURSING: *Making the Most of Mentoring in a Nutshell*, Vance

Fast Facts for DEVELOPING A NURSING ACADEMIC PORTFOLIO: *What You Really Need to Know in a Nutshell*, Wittmann-Price

Fast Facts for the CLASSROOM NURSING INSTRUCTOR: *Classroom Teaching in a Nutshell*, Yoder-Wise, Kowalski

Forthcoming FAST FACTS Books

Fast Facts for the OPERATING ROOM NURSE: *An Orientation and Care Guide in a Nutshell*, Criscitelli

Fast Facts for the LONG-TERM CARE NURSE: *A Guide for Nurses in Nursing Homes and Assisted Living Settings*, Eliopoulos

Fast Facts for the ONCOLOGY NURSE: *Oncology Nursing Orientation in a Nutshell*, Lucas

Fast Facts for the TRIAGE NURSE: *An Orientation and Care Guide in a Nutshell*, Montejano, Grossman

Visit www.springerpub.com to order.

Acknowledgments

We would like to thank God for providing us with the opportunity and resources to nurse and teach.

A special thank you to our editor, Elizabeth Nieginski, and the staff at Springer Publishing Company.

We would like to acknowledge the work of Dr. Diana L. Robins for her kindness in allowing the use of her Modified Checklist for Autism in Toddlers, Revised (M-CHAT-R/F™). What a great screening tool.

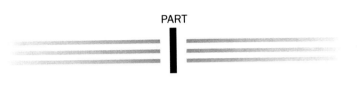

PART

I

Pediatric Principles

Tips for Working With Children

Even if you love children, working with the pediatric population can be tough. First and foremost, the nurse must remember that the child is an essential member of the family and nursing care will be most effective when the entire family is included in the plan of care. Next, the nurse must realize that children are not small adults but special individuals with unique needs. Some differences when working with children and their families include:

- *A pregnancy and birth history, nutritional history, developmental history, habits, and family composition are documented in the assessment.*
- *Assessment techniques do not always progress along a head-to-toe progression; painful or traumatic areas are always assessed last.*
- *Children are not always able to understand why a procedure needs to be done; keep instructions simple*
- *Children yell, cry, and beg when afraid; this can be difficult for novice nurses.*
- *Parents have anxiety and guilt related to the child's illness and hospitalization.*

For all of these reasons, it is important for the pediatric nurse to possess knowledge of normal growth and development as well as a good understanding of the disease disorders common to children. The nurse needs to be organized, calm, and fast. Pediatric nursing is a specialized branch of nursing that is filled with challenges, surprises, and rewards.

This chapter reviews:

1. Strategies on how to relate to pediatric clients
2. Methods that invoke cooperation with pediatric procedures
3. Tips to reduce anxiety in the client and family

APPROACH AND COMMUNICATION

The approach by a nurse when entering a pediatric client's room and the communication that follows depend on the age of the client. The impression the nurse gives during the initial contact, whether good or bad, can impact the child's adjustment to the hospital.

FAST FACTS in a NUTSHELL

The role of the pediatric nurse is threefold:

- A teacher
- A child advocate
- A preventive health provider

GENERAL OVERVIEW FOR INITIAL CONTACT WITH A PEDIATRIC CLIENT

- Greet the child by name.
- Introduce yourself, staff, and roommate, if applicable.
- Provide a tour of the unit or room; point out likeness of room to home, not differences.
- While performing assessment and/or treatment procedures, be matter-of-fact in giving directions.
- Do not rush; calmness is catching.
- Always project a nonjudgmental attitude; the success of the interaction between the nurse and the parents depends on it.
- Avoid discussing details around the pediatric client; step out of the room when discussing medications, treatments, or further testing for younger children.

Infant-Specific Information

- When approaching an infant, address the parent first. If the parent interacts positively with the nurse, the infant will be more accepting.
- Auscultate lungs, heart, and abdomen first; use distraction by handing the infant a block or other toy to keep the infant's attention away from what the nurse is doing.
- Ask the parent to bring in a transitional item such as a favorite toy or blanket. Playing with a familiar item may decrease stress and provide an opening to establish communication.
- Infants have little need for instruction before a procedure. Prepare all equipment before obtaining the child; use the treatment room, not the safe place of the infant's bed.
- Infants between 6 and 30 months exhibit separation anxiety, which is normal. If the infant shows signs of denial, that is a late sign of perceived abandonment.
- An infant's cry is important to note. While a lusty cry is normal, a high-pitched cry can indicate a neurological problem or pain.

FAST FACTS in a NUTSHELL

Parents know their child best. Listen to parental concerns.

Toddler-Specific Information

- The parent is the most important person to the client; keep the toddler and parent together as much as possible and allow parents to be directly involved in care.
- Use minimal contact initially; allow the parent to hold the child on his or her lap. Praise cooperation.
- Keep directions simple and straightforward; language development is limited.
- Do not ask yes or no questions; a toddler's favorite word is "No."
- Behavioral changes are common (regressing, clinging, bed-wetting); these changes are temporary and will diminish once stress levels decrease.

Preschool-Specific Information

- Preschoolers are generally able to explain how they feel; establishing a rapport is important to obtain client cooperation.
- Preschoolers are interested in nurse and doctor roles; this experience may lead to a future occupation.
- Make up a story; children become interested and forget what the nurse is doing.
- Give appropriate choices, which help the child feel a sense of control.
- Demonstrate assessment techniques or procedures on parents or dolls to decrease fear.

School-Age–Specific Information

- These clients are very curious about nursing activities and equipment; allow the client to handle equipment such as a stethoscope or blood pressure cuff and explain the rationale for procedures.
- The child is able to provide specific data on sites and feelings and is able to participate in own care.
- Allow the child to wear underpants and gown; modesty is important. Genitalia is assessed last.
- May develop a crush or look admiringly on the nurse; many children see the nurse as a role model.
- Do not assume that the child understands medical terminology; use simple and common terms (e.g., bowel movement versus poop).

Adolescent-Specific Information

- During assessment, expose only what is to be examined; maintain privacy.
- Explain procedure and rationale before doing; keep the client informed.
- Peers are most important to this age group; allow friends to call or visit, if possible.
- Greatest fear is loss of control in front of peers.
- May mask or deny pain in an effort to be discharged home more quickly.

- Will not admit to a lack of knowledge; ask the client to restate instructions to ensure an understanding.
- Speak matter-of-factly about sexual development or when assessing for drug and alcohol use.
- Emphasize normalcy in physical development.

SUMMARY

The nurse should remember that when a child is hospitalized, the entire family is affected. The parents often experience quilt feelings, blaming themselves for child's illness. The parent and child may also have fears such as the unknown, improper care, financial burden, siblings contracting the disease, and/or the child's potential suffering. The truth is less frightening, but avoid becoming too technical and keep the information age appropriate. The hospital admission can be a distressing time but the nurse can help to make the experience a more pleasant one by being understanding to the parents and the child.

REFERENCES AND FURTHER READING

Hockenberry, M., & Wilson, D. (2013). *Wong's essentials of pediatric nursing* (9th ed.). St. Louis, MO: Elsevier.

Kyle, T., & Carman, S. (2013). *Essentials of pediatric nursing* (2nd ed.). Philadelphia, PA: Wolters Kluwer.

Leifer, G. (2011). *Introduction to maternity & pediatric nursing* (6th ed.). St. Louis, MO: Elsevier.

2

Growth and Development

Growth and development are often referred to as a single unit, as the processes are interrelated throughout infancy to childhood and adolescence. The periods of the most rapid cellular growth occur in utero, during infancy, and in adolescence. Growth refers to an increase in physical size while development refers to the sequential process by which various skills and functions are learned. Maturation refers to an increase in competence and adaptability.

This chapter reviews:

1. Trends in growth and development
2. Developmental stages and milestones
3. Developmental warning signs

PATTERNS OF GROWTH AND DEVELOPMENT

There are definite and predictable patterns of growth and development that allow the nurse to interpret age-appropriate norms. When evaluating, realize that the patterns of growth are symmetrical and bilateral.

These patterns of growth and development include:

- Cephalocaudal or head-to-tail directional growth
- Proximodistal or near-to-far development (i.e., use of arms, then hands, then fingers)

- Sequential trends with a definite pattern (e.g., crawl, creep, stand, walk)
- Differentiation (i.e., a simple operation to more complex operations)

INFLUENCES ON GROWTH AND DEVELOPMENT

Although there are several factors that influence growth and development, one of the most important is nutrition. Children's appetites fluctuate during growth spurts and plateaus. Adequate nutrition is closely related to good health throughout life. Breast and bottle feeding with iron-fortified formulas are the only source of nutrition for the newborn until 4 to 6 months of age when solid foods are introduced into the diet. The typical food progression is cereal, fruit, vegetables, and meat, with a new food introduced every 3 to 5 days.

Parental care, love, and attention also affect growth and development. A nurturing environment, which allows the child to explore the environment, enables the child to meet physical and psychosocial developmental milestones. Without this, the child is at risk for a diagnosis of "failure to thrive," in which the child does not meet height and weight standards, or falls behind in physical, social, and emotional skills.

There are limited times during the process of growth and development of a child when a child interacts with the environment in a specific manner. Called sensitive periods, if the child does not accomplish specific tasks at specific times, the child may be held at that period and be unable to progress.

INFANT (BIRTH TO 1 YEAR OF AGE)

- Weight doubles in 6 months.
- Weight triples and length increases by 50% by 1 year.

Gross motor skills develop in a cephalocaudal fashion as the infant learns to lift the head independently, then roll over, then sit with limited support. Fine motor skills develop in a proximodistal fashion as the infant uses the whole hand to grab objects and then progresses to using the pincer grasp.

Age	Gross Motor Skills	Fine Motor Skills	Language
1–2 months	Lifts and turns head to side, then raises head. Head lags when pulled to sitting	Fists clenched, general or involuntary movements	Cries when needs are not met, makes other vocalizations, coos
3–4 months	Maintains raised head longer, looks around, rolls over, head leads when pulled to a sitting position	Begins to touch objects, unable to grasp them	Laughs aloud, responds to name
5–6 months	Rolls over, sits upright when supported	Grasps and releases objects	Reflects emotions of others, says "no!" personality traits noted
7–8 months	Sits without support or alone	Transfers objects from one hand to another	Babbles, states "mama, dada"
9–10 months	Crawls on hands and knees, pulls to standing position, takes a few steps	Pincer grasp	Imitates others' words and begins to attach meaning, such as "drink"
11–12 months	Sits from standing position, walks	Uses pincer grasp for finger foods	Uses 2–4 recognizable words, some words have specific meaning

FAST FACTS in a NUTSHELL

Medication administration tip!
Liquid medications are calculated for a safe dose (to the hundredth), are prepared in a syringe, and squirted along the side of the mouth.

TODDLER (AGES I TO 3 YEARS)

- Physical growth slows. Average weight 27 pounds, average height 34 inches.
- Birth weight is quadrupled by 2½ years of age; appears potbellied.
- Most important, a child should steadily increase in height and weight.

The rate of acquiring new skills for the toddler declines and the toddler works on refining motor skills, such as standing and walking. Focus of development is on cognitive growth and learning language skills.

Age	Gross Motor Skills	Fine Motor Skills	Language
12–15 months	Walks independently, stretches to reach for objects	Feeds self, points, plays basic games such as tossing an object, gestures	Responds to common words, vocal imitation, uses one-word sentences
18 months	Climbs stairs with assistance, runs but falls easily, masters reaching, grasping, and releasing	Throws a ball overhand, turns pages in a book, assists with dressing and removes shoes and socks	Bilingual children achieve language milestone in two languages simultaneously, increased level of comprehension is noted
24 months	Walks up and down stairs, climbs up and down furniture, improved coordination	Uses both hands to build a tower, uses blocks, scribbles on paper, turns knobs	Word usages increases to approximately 300 words, two-word sentences, asks "why?" questions
30 months	Jumps using both feet, tiptoes	Draws big circles on paper, imitates parents' work using tools	65% of speech is understandable, 2- to 4-word sentences
36 months	Stands on one foot, climbs stairs with alternating feet	Undresses self, runs easily, some details on drawing noted	Acquires 5–6 new words daily, uses polite grammar, uses pronouns

Guidance is provided to parents to identify when a child is ready for toilet training. There are several factors that are helpful to determine readiness for toilet training, such as:

- Anal and urethral sphincter control
- Decreased number of wet diapers/day
- Recognizes urge to defecate or urinate
- Expresses willingness to please parent
- Curiosity of others' toileting habits
- Verbally indicates when wet or soiled

PRESCHOOLER (AGES 3 TO 5 YEARS)

- Rate of physical growth stabilizes
  - Average weight gain 2 to 3 kg/year; average height gain 2.5 to 3.5 inches/year
  - Appearance is slender

During the preschool ages, motor development consists of increases in strength and refinement of previously learned skills. Good posture, appropriate amounts of exercise, and an adequate nutritional intake are essential for growth. Magical thinking is most prevalent during this period.

Age	Gross Motor Skills	Fine Motor Skills	Language
3 years	Walking, running, climbing, and jumping are well established	Improvement of eye/hand coordination, begins writing letters, feeds self once food is prepared	Strings multiple words together to express ideas
4 years	Skips and hops proficiently on one foot, moves forward/backward with ease, kicks ball forward	Draws a person with 2–4 body parts, uses scissors, laces shoes, dresses/undresses without assistance	Speaks in complete sentences, is inquisitive, stays on topic of conversation, vocabulary of 1,500 words
5 years	Skips on alternate feet, skates and swims independently	Handedness is established, prints some letters such as those in name, draws person with 6 body parts	Participates in adult conversations, can count to 10, can retell a story, vocabulary of 2,100 words

FAST FACTS in a NUTSHELL

How should a nurse respond to a child who has strong beliefs due to magical thinking? It is important for the nurse to understand that preschoolers are egocentric as they believe that their thoughts are all powerful and can enable cause/effect circumstances. It is important to stress to preschoolers that thoughts cannot make actions occur. This can relieve the child of guilt feelings for his or her thoughts. Also, the nurse must stress that it is important to state that actions are bad but not the child.

SCHOOL AGE (AGES 6 TO 12 YEARS)

- A time of slow, progressive physical growth
- Amount of calories needed decreases; however, appetite increases
- Little difference between girls and boys in size early on, then girls surpass boys in both weight and height toward the end of this period

School-age children are more graceful and less clumsy on their feet. The children are busy with physical activity of climbing, bicycle riding, and sports. Boys and girls double their strength with a gradual increase in poise and physical skill as well. Typically, girls enter puberty (at 9 to 10 years) earlier than boys (at 10 to 11 years).

Age	Gross Motor Skills	Fine Motor Skills	Language
6–7 years	Enjoys physical activity associated with organized sports; follows coaching/parental directions, which improve coordinated actions; able to throw balls toward a target with some accuracy	Due to increased fine motor skills, artistic interpretations improve, independent use of specialized equipment for oral care and hygiene	Communicates ideas and activities from school to parents, discussion encourages language development

(continued)

Age	Gross Motor Skills	Fine Motor Skills	Language
8–9 years	Honing gross motor skills, able to note a special ability in certain physical activities such as dance or sports, movement fluid	Able to include small, detail-orientated additions to artwork/ceramics, uses tableware, assists with household chores	More confident in participation in adult conversation, able to independently answer questions, learns appropriate grammar
10–12 years	Continued refinement of gross motor skills; strength increases, allowing for more accuracy; plays with pets	More motivated to complete tasks, uses tools for repair, assists with cooking	Participates in communicating group ideas for presentations

FAST FACTS in a NUTSHELL

School-age children exhibit signs of stress in the following common ways:

- Headaches
- Stomachaches/change in eating
- Nightmares/difficulty sleeping
- Regressive behaviors
- Change in behavior/ academic performance

ADOLESCENT (AGES 12 TO 20 YEARS)

- The final 20% to 25% of height is achieved.
- Enlargement of the larynx and vocal cords occurs in males and females to produce voice changes.
- Sexual maturation can be followed in Tanner stages.

Adolescence is a time of growth and development, with body changes in body size and proportion. Sexual characteristics develop as the adolescent reaches sexual maturity. Increased calories and iron, calcium, and zinc are needed for growth.

Age	Gross Motor Skills	Fine Motor Skills	Language
Early adolescence (11–14 years)	Coordination may be impaired due to growth spurts, development of endurance	Increased ability to manipulate objects, improved dexterity used for technical skills and handwriting	Increased communication with proper grammar and parts of speech
Middle adolescence (14–16 years)	Speed and accuracy increase, coordination improves	Hand/eye coordination is fully developed	Able to provide a presentation independently
Late adolescence (17–20 years)	Adult mobility and actions, competitiveness	Precise hand/eye coordination is used for occupational activities	Skills compared with those of adults

FAST FACTS in a NUTSHELL

It is important to understand normal development to be able to assess and identify abnormal development. Though providing a table of norms is helpful in categorizing development, do not fall into the pitfall of comparing your own child, a niece, or nephew to the standard. Always remember that each child develops at his or her own rate.

REFERENCES AND FURTHER READING

Hockenberry, M., & Wilson, D. (2013). *Wong's essentials of pediatric nursing* (9th ed.). St. Louis, MO: Elsevier.

Kyle, T., & Carman, S. (2013). *Essentials of pediatric nursing* (2nd ed.). Philadelphia, PA: Wolters Kluwer.

Leifer, G. (2011). *Introduction to maternity & pediatric nursing* (6th ed.). St. Louis, MO: Elsevier.

3

Well Child Care: Immunizations

Well child care is a continuous process, as is the growth and development of the child. The nurse needs to understand that there are three components to well child care: immunizations, preventive care, and counseling with anticipatory guidance for safety.

This chapter reviews:

1. Recommended immunization schedule for children of all ages
2. Catch-up schedule for children from birth to age 18 years
3. Considerations on immunization for high-risk children

IMMUNIZATIONS

The widespread use of immunizations has been one of the most significant advances in pediatrics and is responsible for the marked decline of preventable diseases. The recommended primary schedule begins in early infancy and is completed during early childhood, with the exception of boosters. Therefore, well child care should include a discussion of childhood immunizations for diphtheria, tetanus, pertussis, poliovirus, measles, mumps, rubella, *Haemophilus influenzae* type b, hepatitis A and B viruses, influenza, rotavirus, chickenpox, and vaccines that protect against meningococcal and pneumococcal infections.

FAST FACTS in a NUTSHELL

> Any immunization may cause an anaphylactic reaction. Epinephrine 1:1000 should be available.

Schedule for Immunizations

In the United States, the Advisory Committee on Immunization Practices (ACIP) of the Centers for Disease Control and Prevention (CDC) and the Committee on Infectious Diseases of the American Academy of Pediatrics govern the recommendations for immunization policies and procedures. In Canada, recommendations are from the National Advisory Committee on Immunization under the authority of the Minister of Health and Public Health Agency of Canada. The policies of each committee are recommendations, not rules, and they change as a result of advances in the field of immunology.

Nurses need to keep informed of the latest advances and changes in policy.

FAST FACTS in a NUTSHELL

> A vaccine series does not need to be restarted, regardless of the time that has elapsed between doses.

For the most current recommended schedules for children, the CDC website can be accessed at: www.cdc.gov/vaccines/schedules/hcp/child-adolescent.html

Recommended Immunization Schedule for Persons Age 0 Through 18 Years

For those whose immunization schedules fall behind or start late, provide catch-up vaccination at the earliest opportunity as indicated by the dark bars in Figure 3.1. To determine minimum intervals between doses, see the catch-up schedule (Figure 3.2).

FIGURE 3.1 Birth to 15 Months

Vaccine	Birth	1 month	2 months	4 months	6 months	9 months	12 months	15 months
Hepatitis B (HepB)	←1st dose→	←2nd dose→			←3rd dose→			
Rotavirus (RV) RV1 (2-dose series); RV5 (3-dose series)			←1st dose→	←2nd dose→				
Diphtheria, tetanus, and acellular pertussis (DTaP: < 7 years)			←1st dose→	←2nd dose→	←3rd dose→			←4th dose→
Tetanus, diphtheria, and acellular pertussis (Tdap: ≥ 7 years)								
Haemophilus influenzae type b (Hib)			←1st dose→	←2nd dose→			←3rd or 4th dose→	
Pneumococcal conjugate (PCV13)			←1st dose→	←2nd dose→	←3rd dose→		←4th dose→	
Pneumococcal polysaccharide (PPSV23)								
Inactivated poliovirus (IPV) (< 18 years)			←1st dose→	←2nd dose→	←3rd dose→			

(continued)

FIGURE 3.1 Birth to 15 Months *(continued)*

Vaccine	Birth	1 month	2 months	4 months	6 months	9 months	12 months	15 months
Influenza (IIV; LAIV) 2 doses for some					Annual vaccination (IIV only)			
Measles, mumps, rubella (MMR)							←1st dose→	
Varicella (VAR)							←1st dose→	
Hepatitis A (HepA)							←2-dose series	
Human papillomavirus (HPV2: females only; HPV4: males and females)								
Meningococcal (Hib-Men-CY ≥ 6 weeks; MenACWY-D ≥ 9 months; MenACWY-CRM ≥ 2 months)								

FIGURE 3.2 18 Months to 18 Years

Vaccines	18 months	19–23 months	2–3 years	4–6 years	7–10 years	11–12 years	13–15 years	16–18 years
Hepatitis B (HepB)	←3rd dose→							
Rotavirus (RV) RV1 (2-dose series); RV5 (3-dose series)								
Diphtheria, tetanus, and acellular pertussis (DTaP: < 7 years)	←4th dose→			←5th dose→				
Tetanus, diphtheria, and acellular pertussis (Tdap: ≥ 7 years)						(Tdap)		
Haemophilus influenzae type b (Hib)								
Pneumococcal conjugate (PCV13)								
Pneumococcal polysaccharide (PPSV23)								
Inactivated poliovirus (IPV; < 18 years)	←3rd dose→			←4th dose→				

(continued)

FIGURE 3.2 18 Months to 18 Years (continued)

Vaccines	18 months	19–23 months	2–3 years	4–6 years	7–10 years	11–12 years	13–15 years	16–18 years
Influenza (IIV; LAIV) 2 doses for some	Annual vaccination (IIV only)	Annual vaccination (IIV or LAIV)						
Measles, mumps, rubella (MMR)				←2nd dose→				
Varicella (VAR)				←2nd dose→				
Hepatitis A (HepA)	←2 dose series							
Human papillomavirus (HPV2: females only; HPV4: males and females)						←(3 dose series)→		
Meningococcal (Hib-Men-CY ≥ 6 weeks; MenACWY-D ≥ 9 months; MenACWY-CRM ≥ 2 months)						←1st dose→		Booster

Hepatitis B (HepB) Vaccine

At Birth

- Administer monovalent HepB vaccine to all newborns before hospital discharge.
- For infants born to hepatitis B surface antigen (HBsAg)–positive mothers, administer HepB vaccine and 0.5 mL of hepatitis B immune globulin (HBIG) within 12 hours of birth. These infants should be tested for HBsAg and antibody to HBsAg (anti-HBs) 1 to 2 months after completion of the HepB series and at age 9 through 18 months.
- If mother's HBsAg status is unknown, within 12 hours of birth administer HepB vaccine. For infants weighing less than 2,000 g, administer HBIG in addition to HepB within 12 hours of birth. Determine mother's HBsAg status as soon as possible and, if she is HBsAg-positive, also administer HBIG for infants weighing 2,000 g or more (no later than age 7 days).

Doses Following the Birth Dose

- The second dose should be administered at age 1 or 2 months. Monovalent HepB vaccine should be used for doses administered before age 6 weeks.
- Infants who did not receive a birth dose should receive three doses of a HepB-containing vaccine on a schedule of 0, 1 to 2 months, and 6 months starting as soon as feasible. See catch-up schedule.
- Administer the second dose 1 to 2 months after the first dose (minimum interval of 4 weeks), administer the third dose at least 8 weeks after the second dose AND at least 16 weeks after the first dose. The final (third or fourth) dose in the HepB vaccine series should be administered no earlier than age 24 weeks.
- Administration of a total of 4 doses of HepB vaccine is recommended when a combination vaccine containing HepB is administered after the birth dose.

Catch-Up Vaccination

- Unvaccinated persons should complete a three-dose series.
- A 2-dose series (doses separated by at least 4 months) of adult formulation Recombivax HB is licensed for use in children aged 11 through 15 years.

Rotavirus (RV) Vaccines

- Minimum age is 6 weeks for both RV-1 [Rotarix] and RV-5 [RotaTeq]).
- Administer a series of RV vaccine to all infants as follows:
  1. If RV-1 is used, administer a two-dose series at 2 and 4 months of age.
  2. If RV-5 is used, administer a three-dose series at ages 2, 4, and 6 months.
  3. If any dose in the series was RV-5 or if vaccine product is unknown for any dose in the series, a total of three doses of RV vaccine should be administered.

Catch-Up Vaccination

- The maximum age for the first dose in the series is 14 weeks, 6 days.

FAST FACTS in a NUTSHELL

The rotavirus vaccine is not given once the child reaches 8 months of age.

Diphtheria and Tetanus Toxoids and Acellular Pertussis (DTaP) Vaccine

- Minimum age for first dose is 6 weeks; exception: DTaP-IPV (Kinrix), 4 years.
- Administer a five-dose series of DTaP vaccine at ages 2, 4, 6, 15 to 18 months, and 4 through 6 years. The fourth dose may be administered as early as age 12 months, provided at least 6 months have elapsed since the third dose.

Catch-Up Vaccination

- The fifth dose of DTaP vaccine is not necessary if the fourth dose was administered at age 4 years or older.

FAST FACTS in a NUTSHELL

When giving DTaP, Hib, and Hep B vaccines simultaneously, give the most reactive vaccine (DTaP) in a separate leg.

Tetanus and Diphtheria Toxoids and Acellular Pertussis (Tdap) Vaccine

- Minimum age is 10 years for Boostrix, 11 years for Adacel.
- Administer one dose of Tdap vaccine to all adolescents aged 11 through 12 years.
- Tdap can be administered regardless of the interval since the last tetanus and diphtheria toxoid-containing vaccine.
- Administer one dose of Tdap vaccine to pregnant adolescents during each pregnancy (preferred during 27 through 36 weeks gestation) regardless of time since prior Td or Tdap vaccination.

Catch-Up Vaccination

- Persons aged 7 years and older who are not fully immunized with DTaP vaccine should receive Tdap vaccine as one (preferably the first) dose in the catch-up series; if additional doses are needed, use Td vaccine. For children 7 through 10 years who receive a dose of Tdap as part of the catch-up series, an adolescent Tdap vaccine dose at age 11 through 12 years should NOT be administered. Td should be administered instead 10 years after the Tdap dose.
- Persons aged 11 through 18 years who have not received Tdap vaccine should receive a dose followed by tetanus and diphtheria toxoids (Td) booster doses every 10 years thereafter.
- An inadvertent dose of DTaP vaccine administered to children aged 7 through 10 years can count as part of the catch-up series. This dose can count as the adolescent Tdap dose, or the child can later receive a Tdap booster dose at age 11 to 12 years.
- If administered inadvertently to an adolescent aged 11 through 18 years, the dose should be counted as the adolescent Tdap booster.

Haemophilus influenzae Type b (Hib) Conjugate Vaccine

- Minimum age is 6 weeks for PRP-T (ACTHIB), DTaP-IPV/Hib (Pentacel) and Hib-MenCY (MenHibrix), PRP-OMP (PedvaxHIB or COMVAX), 12 months for PRP-T (Hiberix).
- Administer a two- or three-dose Hib vaccine primary series and a booster dose (dose 3 or 4 depending on vaccine used

in primary series) at age 12 through 15 months to complete a full Hib vaccine series.

- The primary series with ActHIB, MenHibrix, or Pentacel consists of three doses and should be administered at 2, 4, and 6 months of age. The primary series with PedvaxHib or COMVAX consists of two doses and should be administered at 2 and 4 months of age; a dose at age 6 months is not indicated.
- One booster dose (dose 3 or 4 depending on the vaccine used in primary series) of any Hib vaccine should be administered at age 12 through 15 months. An exception is Hiberix vaccine. Hiberix should only be used for the booster (final) dose in children aged 12 months through 4 years who have received at least one prior dose of Hib-containing vaccine.

Catch-Up Vaccination

- If dose 1 was administered at ages 12 to 14 months, administer booster (as final dose) at least 8 weeks after dose 1, regardless of the Hib vaccine used in the primary series.
- If the first two doses were PRP-OMP (PedvaxHIB or Comvax), and were administered at age 11 months or younger, the third (and final) dose should be administered at age 12 through 15 months and at least 8 weeks after the second dose.
- If the first dose was administered at age 7 through 11 months, administer the second dose at least 4 weeks later and a final dose at age 12 through 15 months or 8 weeks after second dose, whichever is later, regardless of Hib vaccine used for first dose.
- If the first dose is administered at younger than 12 months of age and second dose is given between 12 and 14 months of age, a third (and final) dose should be given 8 weeks later.
- For unvaccinated children aged 15 months or older, administer only one dose.

Vaccination of Persons With High-Risk Conditions

- Children aged 12 through 59 months who are at increased risk for Hib disease, including chemotherapy recipients and those with anatomic or functional asplenia (including sickle cell disease), human immunodeficiency virus (HIV) infection, immunoglobulin deficiency, or early component complement deficiency, who have received either no doses or only one dose of Hib vaccine before 12 months of age, should receive two additional doses of Hib vaccine 8 weeks apart; children who received two or more doses of Hib vaccine before 12 months of age should receive one additional dose.

- For patients younger than 5 years of age undergoing chemotherapy or radiation treatment who received a Hib vaccine dose(s) within 14 days of starting therapy or during therapy repeat the dose(s) at least 3 months following therapy completion.
- Recipients of hematopoietic stem cell transplant (HSCT) should be revaccinated with a three-dose regimen of Hib vaccine starting 6 to 12 months after successful transplant, regardless of vaccination history; doses should be administered at least 4 weeks apart.
- A single dose of any Hib-containing vaccine should be administered to unimmunized* children and adolescents 15 months of age and older undergoing an elective splenectomy; if possible, the vaccine should be administered at least 14 days before procedure.
- Hib vaccine is not routinely recommended for patients 5 years or older. However, one dose of Hib vaccine should be administered to unimmunized* persons aged 5 years or older who have anatomic or functional asplenia (including sickle cell disease) and unvaccinated persons 5 through 18 years of age with human immunodeficiency virus (HIV) infection.

PNEUMOCOCCAL VACCINES

- Minimum age is 6 weeks for PCV13, 2 years for PPSV23.

Routine Vaccination With PCV13

- Administer a four-dose series of PCV13 vaccine at ages 2, 4, and 6 months and at age 12 through 15 months.
- For children ages 14 through 59 months who have received an age-appropriate series of 7-valent PCV (PCV7), administer a single supplemental dose of 13-valent PCV (PCV13).

---

* Patients who have not received a primary series and booster dose or at least one dose of Hib vaccine after 14 months of age are considered unimmunized.

Catch-Up Vaccination With PCV13

- Administer one dose of PCV13 to all healthy children aged 24 through 59 months who are not completely vaccinated for their age.
- For other catch-up guidance, see Figures 3.3 and 3.4.

Vaccination of Persons With High-Risk Conditions With PCV13 and PPSV23

- All recommended PCV13 doses should be administered prior to PPSV23 vaccination, if possible.
- For children 2 through 5 years of age with any of the following conditions: chronic heart disease (particularly cyanotic congenital heart disease and cardiac failure); chronic lung disease (including asthma if treated with high-dose oral corticosteroid therapy); diabetes mellitus; cerebrospinal fluid leak; cochlear implant; sickle cell disease and other hemoglobinopathies; anatomic or functional asplenia; HIV infection; chronic renal failure; nephrotic syndrome; diseases associated with treatment with immunosuppressive drugs or radiation therapy, including malignant neoplasms, leukemias, lymphomas, and Hodgkin's disease; solid organ transplantation; or congenital immunodeficiency:
  - Administer one dose of PCV13 if three doses of PCV (PCV7 and/or PCV13) were received previously.
  - Administer two doses of PCV13 at least 8 weeks apart if fewer than three doses of PCV (PCV7 and/or PCV13) were received previously.
  - Administer supplemental dose of PCV13 if four doses of PCV7 or other age-appropriate complete PCV7 series was received previously.
  - The minimum interval between doses of PCV (PCV7 or PCV13) is 8 weeks.
  - For children with no history of PPSV23 vaccination, administer PPSV23 at least 8 weeks after the most recent dose of PCV13.
- For children aged 6 through 18 years who have cerebrospinal fluid leak; cochlear implant; sickle cell disease and other hemoglobinopathies; anatomic or functional asplenia;

FIGURE 3.3 Catch-up immunization schedule for persons aged 4 months through 6 years who start late or who are more than 1 month behind: United States, 2014. Always use this table in conjunction with Figures 3.1 and 3.2.

Vaccine	Minimum age for dose 1	Minimum Interval Between Doses			
		Dose 1 to dose 2	Dose 2 to dose 3	Dose 3 to dose 4	Dose 4 to dose 5
Hepatitis B	Birth	4 weeks	8 weeks and at least 16 weeks after first dose; minimum age for the final dose is 24 weeks		
Rotavirus	6 weeks	4 weeks	4 weeks		
Diphtheria, tetanus, and acellular pertussis	6 weeks	4 weeks	4 weeks	6 months	6 months

(continued)

FIGURE 3.3 Catch-up immunization schedule for persons aged 4 months through 6 years who start late or who are more than 1 month behind: United States, 2014. Always use this table in conjunction with Figures 3.1 and 3.2. (continued)

Vaccine	Minimum age for dose 1	Dose 1 to dose 2	Dose 2 to dose 3	Dose 3 to dose 4	Dose 4 to dose 5
		Minimum Interval Between Doses			
Haemophilus influenzae type b	6 weeks	4 weeks if first dose administered at younger than age 12 months; 8 weeks (as final dose) if first dose administered at age 12 through 14 months. No further doses needed if first dose administered at age 15 months or older	4 weeks if current age is younger than 12 months and first dose administered at < 7 months old; 8 weeks and age 12 months through 59 months (as final dose) if current age is younger than 12 months and first dose administered between 7 and 11 months (regardless of Hib vaccine [PRP-T or PRP-OMP] used for first dose); OR if current age is 12 through 59 months and first dose administered at younger than age 12 months; OR first 2 doses were PRP-OMP and administered at younger than 12 months. No further doses needed if previous dose administered at age 15 months or older	8 weeks (as final dose). This dose only necessary for children aged 12 through 59 months who received 3 (PRP-T) doses before age 12 months and started the primary series before age 7 months	

Pneumococcal	6 weeks	4 weeks if first dose administered at younger than age 12 months; 8 weeks (as final dose for healthy children) if first dose administered at age 12 months or older. No further doses needed for healthy children if first dose administered at age 24 months or older	4 weeks if current age is younger than 12 months; 8 weeks (as final dose for healthy children) if current age is 12 months or older. No further doses needed for healthy children if previous dose administered at age 24 months or older	8 weeks (as final dose). This dose only necessary for children aged 12 through 59 months who received 3 doses before age 12 months or for children at high risk who received 3 doses at any age
Inactivated poliovirus	6 weeks	4 weeks	4 weeks	6 months; minimum age 4 years for final dose
Meningococcal	6 weeks	8 weeks		
Measles, mumps, rubella	12 months	4 weeks		
Varicella	12 months	3 months		
Hepatitis A	12 months	6 months		

FIGURE 3.4 Catch-up immunization schedule for persons aged 7 through 18 years who start late or who are more than 1 month behind: United States, 2014. Always use this table in conjunction with Figures 3.1 and 3.2.

Vaccine	Minimum age for dose 1	Minimum Interval Between Doses			
		Dose 1 to dose 2	Dose 2 to dose 3	Dose 3 to dose 4	Dose 4 to dose 5
Tetanus, diphtheria; tetanus, diphtheria, and acellular pertussis	7 years	4 weeks	4 weeks if first dose of DTaP/DT administered at younger than age 12 months; 6 months if first dose of DTaP/DT administered at age 12 months or older and then no further doses needed for catch-up	6 months if first dose of DTaP/DT administered at younger than age 12 months	
Human papillomavirus	9 years	Routine dosing intervals are recommended			
Hepatitis A	12 months	6 months			

Vaccine	Minimum age for dose 1	Dose 1 to dose 2	Dose 2 to dose 3	Dose 3 to dose 4
Hepatitis B	Birth	4 weeks	8 weeks (and at least 16 weeks after first dose)	
Inactivated poliovirus	6 weeks	4 weeks	4 weeks	6 months
Meningococcal	6 weeks	8 weeks		
Measles, mumps, rubella	12 months	4 weeks		
Varicella	12 months	3 months if person is younger than age 13 years; 4 weeks if person is aged 13 years or older		

congenital or acquired immunodeficiencies; HIV infection; chronic renal failure; nephrotic syndrome; diseases associated with treatment with immunosuppressive drugs or radiation therapy, including malignant neoplasms, leukemias, lymphomas, and Hodgkin's disease; generalized malignancy; solid organ transplantation; or multiple myeloma:

- If neither PCV13 nor PPSV23 has been received previously, administer one dose of PCV13 immediately and one dose of PPSV23 at least 8 weeks later.
- If PCV13 has been received previously but PPSV23 has not, administer one dose of PPSV23 at least 8 weeks after the most recent dose of PCV13.
- If PPSV23 has been received but PCV13 has not, administer one dose of PCV13 at least 8 weeks after the most recent dose of PPSV23.

- For children aged 6 through 18 years with chronic heart disease (particularly cyanotic congenital heart disease and cardiac failure), chronic lung disease (including asthma if treated with high-dose oral corticosteroid therapy), diabetes mellitus, alcoholism, or chronic liver disease who have not received PPSV23, administer one dose of PPSV23. If PCV13 has been received previously, then PPSV23 should be administered at least 8 weeks after any prior PCV13 dose.

- A single revaccination with PPSV23 should be administered 5 years after the first dose to children with sickle cell disease or other hemoglobinopathies; anatomic or functional asplenia; congenital or acquired immunodeficiencies; HIV infection; chronic renal failure; nephrotic syndrome; diseases associated with treatment with immunosuppressive drugs or radiation therapy, including malignant neoplasms, leukemias, lymphomas, and Hodgkin's disease; generalized malignancy; solid organ transplantation; or multiple myeloma.

Inactivated Poliovirus Vaccine (IPV)

- Minimum age for first dose is 6 weeks.
- Administer a four-dose series of IPV at ages 2, 4, 6 through 18 months, and 4 through 6 years. The final dose in the series should be administered on or after the fourth birthday and at least 6 months after the previous dose.

Catch-Up Vaccination

- In the first 6 months of life, minimum age and minimum intervals are only recommended if the person is at risk for imminent exposure to circulating poliovirus (i.e., travel to a polio-endemic region or during an outbreak).
- If four or more doses are administered before age 4 years, an additional dose should be administered at age 4 years or older and at least 6 months after the previous dose.
- A fourth dose is not necessary if the third dose was administered at age 4 years or older and at least 6 months after the previous dose.
- If both OPV and IPV were administered as part of a series, a total of four doses should be administered, regardless of the child's current age.
- IPV is not routinely recommended for U.S. residents aged 18 years or older.

Influenza Vaccines

- Minimum age is 6 months for inactivated influenza vaccine (IIV), 2 years for live, attenuated influenza vaccine (LAIV)
  - Administer influenza vaccine annually to all children beginning at age 6 months. For most healthy, nonpregnant persons aged 2 through 49 years, either LAIV or IIV may be used. However, LAIV should NOT be administered to some persons, including (a) those with asthma, (b) children aged 2 through 4 years who had wheezing in the past 12 months, or (c) those who have any other underlying medical conditions that predispose them to influenza complications.
- For children aged 6 months through 8 years:
  - For the 2013 to 2014 season, administer 2 doses (separated by at least 4 weeks) to children who are receiving influenza vaccine for the first time. Some children in this age group who have been vaccinated previously will also need two doses.
- For persons aged 9 years and older:
  - Administer 1 dose.

Measles, Mumps, and Rubella (MMR) Vaccine

- Minimum age for first dose is 12 months.
- Administer a two-dose series of MMR vaccine at age 12 through 15 months and 4 through 6 years. The second dose may be administered before age 4 years, provided at least 4 weeks have elapsed since the first dose.
- Administer one dose of MMR vaccine to infants aged 6 through 11 months before departure from the United States for international travel. These children should be revaccinated with two doses of MMR vaccine, the first at age 12 through 15 months (12 months if the child remains in an area where disease risk is high), and the second dose at least 4 weeks later.
- Administer two doses of MMR vaccine to children aged 12 months and older, before departure from the United States for international travel. The first dose should be administered on or after age 12 months and the second dose at least 4 weeks later.

Catch-Up Vaccination

- Ensure that all school-age children and adolescents have had two doses of MMR vaccine; the minimum interval between the two doses is 4 weeks.

FAST FACTS in a NUTSHELL

Live attenuated virus vaccines like MMR and Varicella should NOT be given to children who are immuno compromised.

Varicella (VAR) Vaccine

- Minimum age is 12 months.
- Administer a two-dose series of VAR vaccine at age 12 through 15 months and 4 through 6 years. The second dose may be administered before age 4 years provided at least 3 months have elapsed since the first dose. If the second dose was administered at least 4 weeks after the first dose, it can be accepted as valid.

Catch-Up Vaccination

- Ensure that all persons aged 7 through 18 years without evidence of immunity have two doses of varicella vaccine. For children aged 7 through 12 years, the recommended minimum interval between doses is 3 months (if the second dose was administered at least 4 weeks after the first dose, it can be accepted as valid); for persons aged 13 years and older, the minimum interval between doses is 4 weeks.

Hepatitis A Vaccine (HepA)

- Minimum age for first dose is 12 months.
- Initiate the two-dose HepA vaccine series for children aged 12 through 23 months; separate the two doses by 6 to 18 months.
- Children who have received one dose of HepA vaccine before age 24 months should receive a second dose 6 to 18 months after the first dose.
- For any person aged 2 years and older who has not already received a HepA vaccine series, two doses of HepA vaccine separated by 6 to 18 months may be administered if immunity against hepatitis A virus infection is desired.

Catch-Up Vaccination

- The minimum interval between the two doses is 6 months.

Special Populations

- Administer two doses of HepA vaccine at least 6 months apart to previously unvaccinated persons who live in areas where vaccination programs target older children, or who are at increased risk for infection. This includes persons traveling to or working in countries that have high or intermediate endemicity of infection; men having sex with men; users of injection and noninjection illicit drugs; persons who work with HAV-infected primates or with HAV in a research laboratory; persons with clotting-factor disorders; persons with chronic liver disease; and persons who anticipate close, personal contact (e.g., household or regular babysitting) with an international adoptee during the first 60 days after arrival in the United States from a country with high or intermediate endemicity. The first dose should be administered as soon as the adoption is planned, ideally 2 or more weeks before the arrival of the adoptee.

Human Papillomavirus (HPV) Vaccines (HPV2 [Cervarix] and HPV4 [Gardisil])

- Minimum age for first dose is 9 years.
- Administer a three-dose series of HPV vaccine on a schedule of 0, 1 to 2, and 6 months to all adolescents aged 11 to 12 years. Either HPV4 or HPV2 may be used for females, and only HPV4 may be used for males.
- Administer the second dose 1 to 2 months after the first dose (minimal interval of 4 weeks), administer the third dose 24 weeks after the first dose and 16 weeks after the second dose (minimum interval of 12 weeks).

Catch-Up Vaccination

- Administer the vaccine series to females (either HPV2 or HPV4) and males (HPV4) at age 13 through 18 years if not previously vaccinated.
- Use recommended routine dosing intervals (see above) for vaccine series catch-up.

Meningococcal Conjugate Vaccines

- Minimum age is 6 weeks for Hib-MenCY (MenHibrix), 9 months for MenACWY-D (Menactra), 2 months for MenACWY-CRM (Menveo).
- Administer a single dose of Menactra or Menveo vaccine at age 11 through 12 years, with a booster dose at age 16 years.
- Adolescents aged 11 through 18 years with human immuno-deficiency virus (HIV) infection should receive a two-dose primary series of Menactra or Menveo with at least 8 weeks between doses.
- For children aged 2 months through 18 years with high-risk conditions, see below.

Catch-Up Vaccination

- Administer Menactra or Menveo vaccine at age 13 through 18 years if not previously vaccinated.
- If the first dose is administered at age 13 through 15 years, a booster dose should be administered at age 16 through 18 years with a minimum interval of at least 8 weeks between doses.
- If the first dose is administered at age 16 years or older, a booster dose is not needed.

Vaccination of Persons With High-Risk Conditions and Other Persons at Increased Risk

- Children with anatomic or functional asplenia (including sickle cell disease):
  - For children younger than 19 months of age, administer a four-dose infant series of MenHibrix or Menveo at 2, 4, 6, and 12 through 15 months of age.
  - For children aged 19 through 23 months who have not completed a series of MenHibrix or Menveo, administer two primary doses of Menveo at least 3 months apart.
  - For children aged 24 months and older who have not received a complete series of MenHibrix or Menveo or Menactra, administer two primary doses of either Menactra or Menveo at least 2 months apart. If Menactra is administered to a child with asplenia (including sickle cell disease), do not administer Menactra until 2 years of age and at least 4 weeks after the completion of all PCV13 doses.
- Children with persistent complement component deficiency:
  - For children younger than 19 months of age, administer a four-dose infant series of either MenHibrix or Menveo at 2, 4, 6, and 12 through 15 months of age.
  - For children 7 through 23 months who have not initiated vaccination, two options exist depending on age and vaccine brand:
    - For children who initiate vaccination with Menveo at 7 months through 23 months of age, a two-dose series should be administered, with the second dose after 12 months of age and at least 3 months after the first dose.
    - For children who initiate vaccination with Menactra at 9 months through 23 months of age, a two-dose series of Menactra should be administered at least 3 months apart.

- For children aged 24 months and older who have not received a complete series of MenHibrix, Menveo, or Menactra, administer two primary doses of either Menactra or Menveo at least 2 months apart.
- For children who travel to or reside in countries in which meningococcal disease is hyperendemic or epidemic, including countries in the African meningitis belt or the Hajj, administer an age-appropriate formulation and series of Menactra or Menveo for protection against serogroups A and W meningococcal disease. Prior receipt of MenHibrix is not sufficient for children traveling to the meningitis belt or the Hajj because it does not contain serogroups A or W.
- For children at risk during a community outbreak attributable to a vaccine serogroup, administer or complete an age- and formulation-appropriate series of MenHibrix, Menactra, or Menveo.

Catch-Up Recommendations for Persons With High-Risk Conditions

- If MenHibrix is administered to achieve protection against meningococcal disease, a complete age-appropriate series of MenHibrix should be administered.
- If the first dose of MenHibrix is given at or after 12 months of age, a total of two doses should be given at least 8 weeks apart to ensure protection against serogroups C and Y meningococcal disease.
- For children who initiate vaccination with Menveo at 7 months through 9 months of age, a two-dose series should be administered, with the second dose after 12 months of age and at least 3 months after the first dose.

ADDITIONAL IMMUNIZATION INFORMATION

- Information on travel vaccine requirements and recommendations is available at wwwnc.cdc.gov/travel/page/vaccinations.htm.
- For vaccination of persons with primary and secondary immunodeficiencies, see Table 13, "Vaccination of Persons With Primary and Secondary Immunodeficiencies," in

General Recommendations on Immunization (ACIP), available at www.cdc.gov/mmwr/preview/mmwrhtml/rr6002a1.htm
- Immunization Schedule for Infants and Children, Canada can be accessed from The Public Health Agency of Canada at www.phac-aspc.gc.ca/im/is-cv/index-eng.php#a.

REFERENCES AND FURTHER READING

Centers for Disease Control and Prevention. (2014). *Advisory Committee on Immunization Practices (ACIP) recommended immunization schedule for persons aged 0 through 18 Years—United States.* Retrieved from http://www.cdc.gov/vaccines/schedules/hcp/child-adolescent.html

Hockenberry, M., & Wilson, D. (2013). *Wong's essentials of pediatric nursing* (9th ed.). St. Louis, MO: Elsevier.

Leifer, G. (2011). *Introduction to maternity & pediatric nursing* (6th ed.). St. Louis, MO: Elsevier.

Public Health Agency of Canada. (n.d.). *Immunization schedules: Recommendations from the National Advisory Committee on Immunization (NACI).* Retrieved from http://www.phac-aspc.gc.ca/im/is-cv/index-eng.php#a

4

Well Child Care: Preventive Care and Anticipatory Guidance

Well child care is a continuous process, as is the growth and development of the child. The nurse needs to understand there are three components to well child care: immunizations, preventive care, and counseling of anticipatory guidance for safety.

This chapter reviews:

1. Ongoing health screenings and physical exams for children of all ages
2. General preventive well child care including nutrition, dental health, and sleep
3. Anticipatory guidance and safety needs specific to each age group during childhood

PREVENTIVE WELL CHILD CARE

Children of all ages should receive ongoing health screenings and preventive care checkups.

FAST FACTS in a NUTSHELL

> Physical exams should be performed at least every 1 to
> 3 months throughout infancy, then at least once every year
> until full grown.

Infant

Nutrition

- First 6 months
  - Human milk most desirable (no need for added vitamins/minerals except iron).
  - Formula is also a good source of nutrition.
  - Cow's milk is NOT considered an acceptable form of complete nutrition for an infant at this age.
- Second 6 months
  - Fluoride supplement may be added (if not in the water supply).
  - May begin to add solid food—cereal, fruits, vegetables, then meat.
  - Only add one new food at a time.
  - Juice may be added but in scant amount. Some research suggests fruit juice has been linked to short stature and/or obesity.
  - Whole milk is not introduced until 1 year of age.

Dental Health

- After 2 months of age, wipe gums daily using moist cloth or rinse with water after feedings.
- May introduce soft, small toothbrush.
- Fluoride encouraged after 6 months of age, only if content in water supply is less than 0.6 ppm.
- Encourage weaning to prevent bottle-mouth caries.

Sleep

- Sleep varies during infancy and among individuals.
- The newborn sleeps 16 to 18 hours per day.
- The infant sleeps 8 to 9 hours per night with naps during the day.

Physical Assessment/Exam

- Usually completed at 2 to 4 weeks, 2 months, 4 months, 6 months, 9 months, and 12 months.

Screenings

- Hemoglobin screening for anemia
- Lead level screening
- The United States has no national policy for genetic disorder screening in the newborn/infant period. Many state laws and voluntary guidelines do exist.
- Screening tests for: PKU, sickle-cell disease, thalassemia, galactosemia, hypothyroidism, maple syrup urine disease, homocystinuria, and cystic fibrosis as recommended by the Centers for Disease Control and Prevention (CDC).

Toddler

Nutrition

- As growth rate decreases, so does appetite.
- Amount of food is not as important as a well-balanced diet. Keep healthy snacks available.
- Fatigue greatly influences appetite.
- Present small portions, finger foods, avoid sweets.
- Dawdles at table and fond of rituals.
- Expect messes. Use unbreakable dishes and small utensils. Keep mealtime pleasant.
- Low-fat milk should not be introduced before 2 years of age.

Dental Health

- Tooth brushing with pea-sized amount of toothpaste.
- Fluoride if appropriate.
- Some dentists like to begin exams by age 3 years.

Sleep

- Ten hours per night with one or two naps during the day.

Physical Assessment/Exam

- Well child physical exams completed at 15 months, 18 months, 24 months, and 30 months of age.

Preschool Age

Nutrition

- Nutritional requirements for preschooler are similar to those of toddler.
- Average daily calorie intake is approximately 1,800 calories per day.
- By age 5 years, saturated fatty acids consumption should be less than 10% of total caloric intake.
- Need 800 mg calcium/day.

Dental Health

- By beginning of preschool years, the eruption of the deciduous teeth is completed and teeth may begin to exfoliate.
- Dental care is essential with routine dental prophylaxis every 6 months.
- Require assistance and supervision with brushing, flossing.
- Fluoride supplements as appropriate.
- Limit sweets to daytime meals when saliva content is high.

Sleep

- Patterns vary. Needs approximately 12 hours sleep per night.
- May not nap.
- Waking during night is not uncommon, related to social factors.
- Sleep problems may arise, such as bedtime fears and sleep terror.

Physical Assessment/Exam

- Well child physical exams completed at least once a year.

School Age

Nutrition

- Caloric needs diminish until growth spurt during adolescence.
- The quality of the child's diet depends on family's pattern of eating.

- Promote well-balanced diet, avoiding fast foods.
- Encourage children to participate in meal planning.

Dental Health

- Six-year molar is first permanent tooth. Primary site for caries due to pits and fissures.
- Sealants (plastic coating) may be applied to provide barrier against bacteria.
- Dental care is essential, with routine dental prophylaxis every 6 months.
- Reinforce brushing and flossing techniques.

Sleep

- Amount of sleep required depends on age, activity level, and state of health.
- At age 5 years, requires 11 hours of sleep per night.
- By age 12 years, requires 9 hours of sleep per night.

Physical Assessment/Exam

- Well child physical exams completed at least once a year.

Screenings

- Scoliosis screening
- Hemoglobin and hematocrit
- Urine for sugar and acetone

Adolescent

Nutrition

- Sometimes skips meals and crash diets.
- Assess for potential eating disorders: overeating, undereating, binging, purging.
- Need balanced meals to accommodate physical growth and activity level.

Dental Health

- Motivating the adolescent to assume dental care may be complicated by rebellion.
- Orthodontic treatments place increased risk for gingivitis and caries.
- Mouth protectors should be used to prevent injuries during contact sports.

Sleep

- Needs 8 to 9 hours sleep per night. Often plays catch up on weekends.
- Needs to slow down; due to rapid growth, fatigues easily.

Physical Assessment/Exam

- Well child physical exams completed at least once a year until adulthood.

ANTICIPATORY GUIDANCE

Childrearing is no easy task. Due to our changing society, parents may look to the nurse for professional guidance. Teaching opportunities will vary for each age group.

Infant

Since injuries are a major cause of death during infancy, safety promotion and injury prevention are the focus during this stage of development.

Aspiration

- Avoid use of powders.
- Never prop bottle.
- Keep small objects (buttons, beads, small toys) out of reach.
- Avoid hard candy, nuts, hotdogs, popcorn, marshmallows, and other choking foods.
- Inspect toys for removable parts.

- Keep toxic substances away from the reach of children.
- Do NOT store toxic substances in food/drink containers.
- Post local poison control center phone number near telephone.
- Know emergency procedures for choking infant.

Suffocation and Drowning

- Keep all plastic bags out of reach.
- Do NOT cover mattress with plastic.
- Use firm mattress, loose blankets, and NO pillows.
- Follow "back to sleep" protocol.
- Make sure crib slats meet federal regulations (2.375 inches apart).
- Do NOT tie pacifier around infant's neck.
- Remove bibs at bedtime.
- Never leave infant alone in bath.
- No beanbag-type seats.
- Keep latex balloons out of reach.
- Remove all hanging crib toys once infant can sit up.
- Fence swimming pool and other bodies of water.
- Be alert to water hazards such as buckets, toilets, or standing water containers.
- Keep bathroom doors closed.

Burns

- Install smoke detectors on all levels of the home.
- Avoid heating formula in the microwave.
- Check bathwater before placing infant in water.
- Keep faucet out of reach.
- Keep hot water heater setting at 120° F or lower.
- Keep electrical wires hidden or out of reach.
- Place guards over electrical outlets.
- Place guards in front of any heating appliance.
- Avoid pouring hot liquids while holding child or when child is close by.
- Limit exposure to sun, apply sunscreen.
- Wash flame-retardant clothing according to label directions.
- Use cool mist vaporizers.
- Do NOT leave child in parked car.
- Do NOT use table cloth.
- Avoid smoking while holding child.

Motor Vehicles

- Transport infant in federally approved, rear-facing car seat.
- Secure car seat system accurately in rear seat.
- Never leave infant unattended in car.
- Never park stroller at the rear of the vehicle.

FAST FACTS in a NUTSHELL

Car seats will have an expiration date printed or embossed on the bottom of the seat and should not be used once expired.

Falls and Bodily Injury

- Always use crib rails.
- Never leave infant unattended on bed, raised surface, or unguarded surface.
- Restrain while in highchair.
- Avoid walkers.
- Fence stairways at top and bottom.
- Ensure furniture is sturdy and will not tip.
- Avoid placing televisions and other large objects on top of unsteady furniture.

Toddler and Preschool Age

In the United States, children ages 1 to 4 years of age have the second-highest rate of death due to accidental injuries. Young children are very curious explorers who climb, crawl, run, touch, smell, taste, and smear everything. They are clumsy and awkward, especially when learning new skills. Young children do not have the understanding and are unable to gauge danger. Many of the prevention techniques listed for the infant will also apply to the toddler and preschool-age child.

Motor Vehicles

- Use federally approved car restraint per manufacturer's recommendation for age and weight.
- Always supervise children while playing outdoors.

- Do not allow child to play on curb or between parked cars.
- Supervise bicycle/tricycle riding and always use helmet.
- Teach pedestrian safety rules.

Drowning

- Supervise closely when near any source of water.
- Never leave unattended in bathtub.
- Fence swimming pools and bodies of water.
- Keep bathroom doors closed.

Burns

- Use back burners and turn pot handles toward back of stove.
- Place electrical appliances on back of counters.
- Place guards in front of any heating appliance.
- Store matches and lighters in locked, secure place.
- Keep burning candles out of reach.
- Do not allow electrical cords to hang within reach.
- Teach what "hot" means.
- Apply sunscreen when exposed to sunlight.

Poisoning

- Place all potentially toxic agents, cleaning solutions, pesticides, and personal care items out of reach.
- Keep house plants out of reach.
- Use child-proof caps on all prescription medications.
- Keep all medications and vitamins out of reach.
- Never store toxic agents in food/fluid containers.

Falls and Bodily Injury

- Use window guards (screens are not secure).
- Place gates at top and bottom of stairs.
- Ensure safe and effective barriers on porches, decks, and balconies.
- Remove unsecured or scatter rugs.
- Apply nonskid bathtub bottom.
- Move child to youth bed when able to climb out of crib.
- Dress in safe clothing and avoid laces on shoes.
- Supervise while at playground or play yard.
- Avoid lollypops with stick handles (unless sitting and supervised).

- Teach safety precautions when handling sharp items.
- Store all dangerous tools, garden equipment, and firearms in a locked cabinet.
- Be alert to danger of unsupervised animals and pets.
- Use safety glass on all openings accessible to children.
- Teach child name, address, and/or sew into clothing.
- Teach stranger danger.

Choking/Suffocation

- Avoid hard candy, nuts, hotdogs, popcorn, marshmallows, and other choking foods.
- Discard old refrigerators with doors removed.
- Change batteries in smoke and carbon monoxide alarms every 6 months.
- Develop a fire escape plan for the entire family and practice drills.
- Keep automatic garage door opener in safe place or install new choke-free system.
- Avoid heavy, hinged-lid toy box.
- Keep window blind cords out of reach.
- Remove drawstring from clothing or limit to 6 inches in length.
- Avoid toys that are small enough to be placed in the mouth.

School Age

Parents of the school-age child share their child's time with peer groups and other adults who are assigned a supervisory role. Injury prevention is directed toward education on play equipment, environment, and sports activities.

Motor Vehicle

- Instruct on proper use of seat belts and sitting in back seat.
- Educate on proper passenger behavior.
- Emphasize safe pedestrian behavior.
- Always use helmet with bicycle and ATV use and replace helmet every 5 years.
- Ride bicycle single file and with traffic.
- Walk bicycle through busy intersections at the crosswalk.

- Keep both hands on handlebars except when signaling.
- Equip bicycle with proper lights and reflectors.
- Never hitch a ride on side of vehicle while on the bicycle.

Drowning

- Teach child how to swim.
- Teach basic water safety rules.
- Select safe and supervised places to swim.
- Teach to swim with a companion.
- Review sufficient water depth for diving.

Burns

- Instruct child in areas involving contact with burn hazards (gasoline, starter fluids, matches, chemistry sets, firecrackers, barbeque grills, bonfires).
- Instruct on avoiding flying kites or climbing near high-tension wires.
- Instruct child on behavior in the event of a fire.
- Instruct on cooking safety and proper use of microwave or oven.

Poisoning

- Educate child on hazards of taking nonprescription drugs, chemicals, and alcohol.
- Teach child to say "NO" to drugs and alcohol.

Bodily Injury

- Help provide access to facilities with supervised activities.
- Encourage play in safe areas.
- Keep firearms in locked cabinet—use only with adult supervision.
- Teach proper, safe use of appliances and tools.
- Teach not to tease dogs or interfere with feeding.
- Teach the use of protective equipment in sports and activities.
- If uses contact lenses, teach proper use and care and need for changing to prevent eye damage or infection.
- Teach stranger safety and avoid personalized clothing in public areas.

Adolescent

Adolescence is a confusing and perplexing time for both the adolescent and his or her parents. Parents need to understand that the adolescent is struggling for independence, has a strong need to belong, and is subject to unpredictable behavior.

Motor Vehicle

- Provide driver education.
- Discourage distracting behaviors such as eating, texting, or cell phone use while driving.
- Teach seat belt use for all passengers.
- No drag racing or speeding.
- Reinforce the dangers of drugs and alcohol when operating a vehicle.
- Promote appropriate passenger behavior while riding in a vehicle, including refusal to ride with an impaired or reckless driver.

Pedestrian

- At night, walk with a friend, take well-traveled walkways, and avoid secluded areas.
- If being followed, go to nearest place with people.

Drowning

- Teach how to swim.
- Teach basic rules: sufficient water depth for diving, selection of places to swim, swimming with a companion, and no alcohol use with water sports.

Burns

- Reinforce proper behavior in areas with burn hazards.
- Teach hazards of artificial tanning.
- Encourage use of sunscreen.
- Discourage smoking.

Poisoning

- Reinforce education on hazards of drugs and alcohol.

Bodily Injury

- Promote instruction in sports and use of proper equipment.
- Instruct in safe use and respect for firearms.
- Be alert to signs of depression.
- Encourage and foster safety principles.

CONCLUSION

During childhood, growth and physical changes are occurring at a rapid pace. It is necessary to provide continuous well child care visits and assessments throughout childhood, even when the child appears healthy.

REFERENCES AND FURTHER READING

Hockenberry, M., & Wilson, D. (2013). *Wong's essentials of pediatric nursing* (9th ed.). St. Louis: Elsevier.

Leifer, G. (2011). *Introduction to maternity & pediatric nursing* (6th ed.). St. Louis: Elsevier.

5

Physical Exam:
Newborn Through Adolescence

The nurse must consider the developmental level of the pediatric patient when planning physical assessment sites and techniques. All physical assessments begin with an inspection of the general appearance. It is important to understand that children cannot always communicate what is wrong. Also, a child may look normal and actually be in distress due to the body's ability to compensate. When no longer able to compensate, the child's condition deteriorates quickly and must be treated aggressively to acquire the best outcome.

The first interaction between the child, family, and the nurse can provide crucial data on the status of the child. If a child is interacting with the parent and interested in the surroundings, the nurse recognizes that the child is not in imminent danger. If the child is listless, has a weak cry, and does not object to nurse assessment or medical interventions, the nurse recognizes that the child is critically ill. Notable characteristics include physical appearance, posture, eye contact, speech/lust of cry, motor skills, and growth. Growth charts can be obtained at www.cdc.gov/growthcharts.

This chapter reviews:

1. Techniques for pediatric physical assessment
2. Unique physical assessment findings related to the pediatric population
3. Methods to gain cooperation by the pediatric patient at various ages

DEVELOPMENTALLY APPROPRIATE APPROACHES TO PHYSICAL ASSESSMENT

- Neonates/infants most often comply with the will of the nurse's physical assessment techniques. The parent provides valuable data on the neonate's status. Neonates are best assessed when they are sleeping or being quiet.
- Toddlers are difficult to assess due to stranger anxiety and separation anxiety from the parent. The best time to assess the toddler is during sleep or in the parent's arms, as the parent can comfort or distract the toddler. When initially approaching the child, speak to the parents first as this demonstrates to the toddler that the nurse is safe.
- The preschooler may be shy or unsure of the nurse. It is best to approach preschoolers at their own level and speak to them and their parents first before proceeding. Play with toy medical equipment can decrease anxiety.
- The school-age child is curious and may admire the nurse. It is important for the nurse to address the child and allow the child to handle equipment or to demonstrate the physical assessment techniques on a doll.
- Adolescents understand that a physical assessment needs completion and complies with the nurse's instructions. Consider modesty issues.

FAST FACTS in a NUTSHELL

The Broselow Tape is a laminated, color-coded, quick reference guide that allows health care personnel to determine proper dosages of medication and/or equipment to be used for the child of a certain height and weight. The nurse places the tape so the red arrow is at the child's head and extends the tape, laying it beside the child, to the feet with the toes pointed upward. The nurse looks at the colored areas noted at the child's feet.

Vital Signs

Temperature

Normal Temperature

Note: Normal rectal for children is 37° to 37.5° C or 98.6° to 99.5° F

The American Academy of Pediatrics recommends the axillary route for infants under 1 month of age

The rectal temperature is contraindicated in infants under 1 month of age, children with diarrhea, children with anorectal lesions, and children receiving chemotherapy

Fever is defined as temperature above 38° C (100.4° F)

Recommended Routes

Birth to 2 years
- Axillary
- Rectal, if definitive temperature reading is needed in infants over 1 month of age. Nursing standard for precise diagnosis of fever in infants and young children

2 to 5 years
- Axillary
- Tympanic
- Oral, when child can hold thermometer under tongue
- Rectal, if definitive temperature reading is needed

Over 5 years
- Oral, most accurate for assessing fever in older child
- Axillary
- Tympanic

Pulse

May use radial in children older than 2 years. Apical pulse more reliable in infant and young child. Count for a full minute in the infant and young child.

Heart Rates (beats/minute)

Age	Resting Awake	Resting Sleeping
Newborn	100–180	90–160
1 week–3 months	100–220	80–200
3 months–2 years	80–150	70–120
2–10 years	70–110	60–90
10 years–adult	55–90	50–90

Respiration Rate

Observe abdomen movements in infants because respirations are primarily diaphragmatic. Count for a full minute because movements may be irregular.

Age	Breaths/Minute
Newborn	36
1–11 months	30
2 years	25
4 years	23
8 years	20
10–12 years	19
14 years	18
16 years	17
18 years	16–18

Normal Blood Pressures (BPs) Are Based on Child's Age and Height Percentile

Normal blood pressure

BP less than 90th percentile is normal. BP between 90th and 95th percentile is prehypertensive. In adolescents, BP of 120/80 or greater is prehypertensive.

Cuff size

Cuff bladder width should be approximately 40% of circumference of arm measured at a point midway between olecranon and acromion. Cuff bladder length should cover 80% to 100% of arm circumference.

In the absence of infants/children being able to provide specific data on their symptoms, vital signs can provide valuable data such as:

- Indications of pain
- Indications of internal hemorrhage
- Indications of impending respiratory distress

It is important that the pediatric nurse has an understanding of normal vital signs so that abnormal vital signs are quickly addressed.

Infant Reflexes

- Reflexes assess neurological function.
- Physical assessment of reflexes begins at birth.

Reflex	Assessment	Age Present
Sucking and rooting	Assessed by stroking an infant's cheek or edge of mouth. Reflex: Infant turns head to side that is touched.	Birth to 4 months
Moro reflex (startle)	Assessed by striking surface near infant. Reflex: The arms and legs are symmetrically extended and then abduct while the fingers form to make a C shape.	Birth to 4 months
Palmar grasp	Assessed by placing an object in the infant's hand. Reflex: Infant grasps the object.	Birth to 3 months
Plantar grasp	Assessed by touching the sole of the infant's foot. Reflex: Infant's toes curl downward.	Birth to 8 months
Tonic neck reflex (fencer position)	Assessed by turning the infant's head to one side. Reflex: The infant extends the arm and leg on that side and flexes the arm and leg on the opposite side.	Birth to 4 months
Babinski reflex	Stroke up the lateral edge and across the edge of the infant's foot to elicit a positive Babinski Reflex: Fanning of the toes.	Birth changes to an adult response by 1–2 years
Stepping reflex	Hold the infant upright under the arms with the feet on a flat surface. Reflex: Regular alternating steps.	Birth to 4 weeks

PHYSICAL ASSESSMENT SEQUENCE

- Utilize your understanding of a complete systematic assessment. The assessment considerations below are general and related to the pediatric population.
- Physical assessment sites and techniques are dependent upon age/developmental stage and activity level.

Assessment Site	Assessment Technique	Considerations
Skin, hair, nails	Inspection	• Skin variations according to race or birth marks, turgor brisk • Hair evenly distributed, lanugo noted on the newborn, sexual maturation with hair distribution • Nails pink, smooth, no clubbing indicating oxygen compromise *Pediatric variation: Mongolian spot is a hyperpigmentation in Black, Asian, American Indian, and Hispanic newborns. It is a black-purple area on the skin that resembles bruises.*
Head and neck	Inspection	• Head symmetrical, fontanels flat • Anterior (diamond shaped) closes in 9 months to 2 years
Eyes	Palpation Inspection via ophthalmoscope	• Posterior (triangle shaped) closes in 1–2 months • Face symmetrical • Neck is short in infants, supple, no palpable masses, full range of motion of neck • Eyes have no drainage, visual acuity difficult to assess under 3 years, Snellen chart used over 3 years, conjunctiva pink, sclera white, PERRLA *Pediatric variation: Bulging fontanels indicate an increase in intracranial pressure.*

(continued)

Assessment Site	Assessment Technique	Considerations
Ears	Inspection	• Ear alignment: 10-degree angle from top of auricle to outer canthus
	Inspection via otoscope	• Cerumen is expected; remove from outer canal • Tympanic membrane pearly pink or gray; hearing grossly intact *Pediatric variation: Assessment of inner ear—infant/toddlers, pull pinna down and back; over 3 years, pull up and back*
Nose	Inspection	• Midline and intact, both nares patent • Mucosa is pink and moist, no drainage *Pediatric variation: A transverse line on the nose is a feature of chronic allergies formed when the child uses the hand to push the nose up and back (the "allergic salute").*
Mouth	Inspection	• Gums pink, against teeth • Lips/mucous membranes pink and moist • Infants may have a white coating on tongue from milk, which is easily wiped away
Teeth	Inspection	• Teeth: 6–8 teeth erupt by 1 year • Teeth should be white and not have black dental caries. Children replace 20 deciduous teeth with 32 permanent teeth
Hard and soft palate	Palpation	• Intact, firm, free of ulcers
Tonsils	Inspection	• Infants: May not be able to visualize • Children: Can be seen in back of throat, same color as mucosa • Tonsillitis: Red and edematous, painful *Pediatric variation: Dental caries are No. 1 chronic disease of childhood; cleft lip/cleft palates cause feeding difficulties until surgical correction.*

(continued)

(continued)

Assessment Site	Assessment Technique	Considerations
Thorax	Inspection	• Chest shape: barrel shaped in infants • Ribs/sternum: symmetrical movement
Lungs	Auscultation	• Movement: symmetrical, no retractions, respirations easy • Infants: irregular respirations are normal • Inspiration longer and louder than expiration • Vesicular or swishing sounds heard throughout lung fields when normal
Breasts	Inspection and palpation	• Neonates have enlarged breasts during the first few days after birth. Nipples and areola are darker pigmented and symmetrical • Females: Breast development between 10–14 years. Symmetrical, no masses or drainage • Males: May develop gynecomastia *Pediatric variation: The infant is an obligatory nose breather until 3 months; count respiratory rate for a full minute; brief periods of apnea less than 10–15 seconds are common.*
Circulatory system	Auscultation	• Heart sounds: S1/S2 should be distinct and heard at the apex. Sinus arrhythmias timed with respirations are common. Physiologic splitting of S2 and S3 is common. Pulses strong and equal
Heart	Palpation	• Infants' pulses: brachial, temporal, femoral
Peripheral pulses		• Children/adolescents' pulses: same as adults *Pediatric variation: The heart's position in the infant's chest is more horizontal, thus the apex is higher at the 4th left intercostal space.*

(continued)

Assessment Site	Assessment Technique	Considerations
Abdomen	Inspection	• No rashes, peristaltic waves may be visible—normal in thin children. No protrusions at umbilicus
	Auscultation	• Bowel sounds heard in all 4 quadrants. Normal rate: 5–30/minute
	Palpation	• Abdomen soft, no masses, nontender • Dullness percussed over the liver
	Percussion	*Pediatric variation: Infants have protruded abdomens; otherwise, children have flat abdomens.*
Male genitalia	Inspection	• Hair distribution is diamond shaped after puberty
	Palpation	• Penis straight, meatus at tip, foreskin removed following circumcision. Enlargement during adolescence • Palpate testes for any masses. Left testicle hangs slightly lower than right
		Pediatric variation: No pubic hair noted on infants and young children.
Female genitalia	Inspection	• Hair distribution noted over mons pubis as puberty approaches. Labia symmetrical • No discharge from urethral meatus or vaginal opening before puberty. Menses may begin as early as 9 years old • Hymen may be present over the vaginal opening prior to having sexual intercourse
		Pediatric variation: No pubic hair noted on infants and young children.

(continued)

(continued)

Assessment Site	Assessment Technique	Considerations
Musculoskeletal system	Inspection	• Arms and legs are symmetrical. Moves all extremities through full range of motion • No crepitus in joints, redness, pain
	Palpation	• Deep tendon reflexes–biceps, triceps, patellar, Achilles *Pediatric variation: Muscle strength increases throughout childhood and with strengthening exercise.*
Spine		• Midline. No scoliosis in adolescents
Gait	Inspection	• Toddlers/preschoolers: Bowlegged or knock-knee is common • Gait unsteady and clumsy until school-age period *Pediatric variation: Balance improves throughout childhood and with practice. Assess the ability to hop on one foot.*
Neurological system		Orientation, alertness, relating to parents, cry reflexes, PERRLA *Pediatric variation: The lustiness and pitch of an infant's cry can provide data about an infant's condition. A high-pitch cry can alert to neurological dysfunction or meningitis and a whimpering cry can alert to infant fatigue.*

PAIN ASSESSMENT

Pain assessment involving children has many obstacles, including age and a lack of understanding and interpretation of pain levels. Many believe that children, especially infants, do not feel pain in the same intensity as adults. Other obstacles include:

• Lack of routine pain assessment
• Lack of knowledge in pain treatment

- Fear of adverse effects of analgesics, especially respiratory depression and addiction
- Belief that preventing pain in children takes too much time and effort

Nurses use different pain scales, appropriate to the child's age and level of understanding, to determine the level of pain in their pediatric clients. The scales are divided into the Behavioral Observation Scales for neonates and infants and the Self-Report Scales for children over 3 years of age.

Behavioral Observation Scales	Description
Neonatal/Infants Pain Scale (NIPS)	The NIPS is a behavioral scale composed of six indicators: • Facial expression • Cry • Breathing pattern • Arms • Legs • State of arousal Scores range from 0–7. Greater or equal to 4 indicates severe pain.
CRIES	Behavior scale composed of five indicators: • Crying • Oxygen Requirement • Increased vital signs • Facial Expression • Sleep Useful for neonatal postoperative pain.
FLACC	Behavior scale composed of five indicators: • Face • Legs • Activity • Crying • Consolability Valid from 2 months–7 years.
CHEOPS	Children's Hospital of Eastern Ontario Scale Assess: • Cry • Facial expression • Verbalization • Torso movement • If child touches affected site • Position of legs Intended for children 1–7 years.

Self-Report Scales for Children 3 Years and Older	Description
Wong-Baker Faces Scale	Six cartoon faces showing degrees of distress Face 0: No hurt Face 5: Worst pain imaginable The child chooses the face that best describes pain.
Bieri-Modified	Six cartoon faces starting from a neutral state and progressing to tears and crying.
Visual Analog Scale	Uses a 10-cm line with one end mark of no pain and the opposite end as the worst pain imaginable. The child is to mark the spot on the continuum that represents the amount of pain. Color may also be added.

FAST FACTS in a NUTSHELL

Parents are the best judge of their child's behavior. When parents state that their child is not acting "like himself or herself," nurses must take that very seriously and ask probing questions to identify what is different about the child's behavior. At no time should a parent's comment be dismissed.

REFERENCES AND FURTHER READING

Centers for Disease Control and Prevention. (2014). *Growth charts.* Retrieved from http://www.cdc.gov/growthcharts

Hockenberry, M., & Wilson, D. (2013). *Wong's essentials of pediatric nursing* (9th ed.). St. Louis, MO: Elsevier.

Jarvis, C. (2012). Physical examination and health assessment. (6th ed.). St. Louis, MO: Elsevier.

Kyle, T., & Carman, S. (2013). Essentials of pediatric nursing (2nd ed.). Philadelphia, PA: Wolters Kluwer.

Leifer, G. (2011). *Introduction to maternity & pediatric nursing* (6th ed.). St. Louis, MO: Elsevier.

6

Child Abuse:
How and When to Report

Child abuse is more than a visible injury and can present in many forms: neglect, physical abuse, emotional abuse, and sexual abuse. Abuse, in any form, can leave deep, lasting scars. The earlier the abused child gets help, the greater the chance for healing and breaking the cycle that may lead to perpetuating further abuse. The nurse who knows the common signs of abuse is in a position to intervene and make a difference in the life of a child.

Child Protective Service Laws have been enacted to provide a system of reporting suspected child abuse. Licensees of the Board of Nursing are charged with the responsibility to report suspected child abuse. Failure to comply can result in disciplinary action by the Professional Nurse Board. All reasonable cause to suspect that a child is an abused child MUST be reported.

This chapter reviews:

1. The definition of abuse according to the Federal Child Abuse Prevention and Treatment Act
2. When to report abuse
3. How to report abuse
4. Cultural issues and perceptions of abuse

Question: Is it considered abuse if there is no apparent violence?

Answer: Physical abuse is just one type of child abuse. Neglect and emotional abuse can be just as damaging, and since they are more subtle, other persons are less likely to intervene.

DEFINITION OF ABUSE

Federal legislation provides guidance to states by identifying a set of acts or behaviors that define child abuse and neglect. The Federal Child Abuse Prevention and Treatment Act (CAPTA) (42 U.S.C.A. § 5106g), as amended by the CAPTA Reauthorization Act of 2010, defines child abuse and neglect as, at minimum:

- "Any recent act or failure to act on the part of a parent or care-taker which results in death, serious physical or emotional harm, sexual abuse, or exploitation"
- "An act or failure to act which presents an imminent risk of serious harm"

A "child" under this definition generally means a person who is younger than age 18 or who is not an emancipated minor (www.acf.hhs.gov/programs/cb/resource/capta2010).

WHEN TO REPORT

A single lesion of impetigo can appear to be a cigarette burn. A severe diaper rash, caused by a fungal infection, may look like a scald burn. Be factual and objective when assessing for signs of possible child abuse.

The nurse is responsible for reporting ANY reasonable cause to suspect child abuse. It is NOT the responsibility of the nurse to investigate or authenticate the abuse prior to reporting. Child abuse is not always obvious. By learning the common warning signs of child abuse and neglect, the nurse may be able to identify the problem, stop the cycle, and provide appropriate treatment for the child.

Warning signs of emotional abuse in children:

- Excessively withdrawn, fearful, or anxious about doing something wrong.
- Shows extremes in behavior (extremely compliant or extremely demanding; extremely passive or extremely aggressive).
- Doesn't seem to be attached to the parent or caregiver.
- Acts either inappropriately adult (taking care of other children) or inappropriately infantile (rocking, thumb sucking, throwing tantrums).

Warning signs of physical abuse in children:

- Frequent injuries or unexplained bruises, welts, or cuts.
- Is always watchful and "on alert," as if waiting for something bad to happen.
- Injuries appear to have a pattern such as marks from a hand or belt.
- Pulls away from touch, flinches at sudden movements, or seems afraid to go home.
- Wears inappropriate clothing to cover up injuries, such as long-sleeved shirts on hot days.

Warning signs of neglect in children:

- Clothes are ill fitting, filthy, or inappropriate for the weather.
- Hygiene is consistently bad (unbathed, matted, and unwashed hair; noticeable body odor).
- Untreated illnesses and physical injuries.
- Is frequently unsupervised or left alone or allowed to play in unsafe situations and environments.
- Is frequently late or missing from school.

Warning signs of sexual abuse in children:

- Trouble walking or sitting.
- Displays knowledge or interest in sexual acts inappropriate to his or her age, or even seductive behavior.
- Makes strong efforts to avoid a specific person, without an obvious reason.
- Doesn't want to change clothes in front of others or participate in physical activities.
- An STI or pregnancy, especially under the age of 14.
- Runs away from home.

Just because you see a warning sign doesn't automatically mean a child is being abused. Initiate the report and let the child welfare system take over.

HOW TO REPORT

Reporting requires a phone call to the state child abuse reporting number.

- The nurse provides the facts to the reporting center. If the information warrants further investigation, Child Protective Services and local police will be notified by the reporting center.
- The nurse may also need to follow the policy for reporting within the facility employed.

The National Childline Reporting Center is available 24 hours at 1-800-422-4453. The national center will take the general report but the nurse needs to know:

- The report should be initiated "where" the abuse occurred. For example, if a child who resides in Ohio is abused while on vacation in Virginia, the report should be filed in Virginia.
- Some states prefer reporting to the county first. Childline volunteers will assist in the details of how to report.

For the most current information on individual states' child abuse reporting numbers, refer to the National Organizations section of Child Welfare Information Gateway at www.childwelfare.gov/organizations/index.cfm.

FAST FACTS in a NUTSHELL

Reporting is anonymous. The child abuser cannot find out who made the report of child abuse.

ANTICIPATORY GUIDANCE: ABUSE RISK FACTORS

While child abuse and neglect occur in all types of families—even in those that look happy from the outside—children are at a much greater risk in certain situations. The nurse can advocate for the child by knowing the risk factors for child abuse and neglect.

Domestic Violence

- Witnessing domestic violence is terrifying to children and emotionally abusive.
- Even if the parent does his or her best to protect children from physical abuse, the situation is still extremely damaging.

Alcohol and Drug Abuse

- Living with an alcoholic or addict is very difficult for children and can lead to abuse and neglect.
- A parent who is drunk or high is unable to care for children, make good parenting decisions, and/or control dangerous impulses.

Untreated Mental Illness

- A parent who suffers from depression, anxiety disorder, bipolar disorder, or another mental illness may have trouble taking care of children.
- A mentally ill or traumatized parent may be distant and withdrawn, or quick to anger.
- Treatment for the caregiver means better care for the children.

Lack of Parenting Skills

- Some caregivers never learned the skills necessary for good parenting.
- Teen parents may have unrealistic expectations about how much care babies and small children need.
- A parent who was a victim of child abuse may only know how to raise children in the same manner.
- Parenting classes, therapy, and caregiver support groups are great resources for learning better parenting skills.

Stress and Lack of Support

- Parenting can be a very time-intensive, difficult job. Lack of support, relationship problems, and/or financial difficulties may add to the burden.
- Caring for a child with a disability, special needs, or difficult behaviors can be a challenge.
- It is important to get the support needed by the family.

CULTURAL ISSUES RELATED TO CHILD ABUSE

Complete a culturally sensitive history. Some cultural practices of folk healing by loving parents can be misinterpreted as abuse. Examples of cultural healing practices may include:

Coining

- A Vietnamese practice that may produce welt-like lesions on the back.
- The edge of a coin is repeatedly rubbed lengthwise on the oiled skin to rid the body of disease.

Cupping

- An old-world practice of placing a container of steam against the skin surface to draw out the poison or other evil element.
- The heated air in the container cools, and a vacuum is created that produces a bruise-like blemish on the skin beneath the mouth of the container.

Burning

- A practice of some Southeast Asian groups where small areas of skin are burned to treat enuresis and temper tantrums.

Female Circumcision

- Removal or mutilation to any part of the female genital organ.
- A practice in Africa, the Middle East, Latin America, India, Asia, North America, Australia, and Western Europe.

Forced Kneeling

- A form of child discipline in some Caribbean groups.

Topical Garlic Application

- A practice of Yemenite Jews in which crushed garlic paste is applied to the wrists to treat infections.
- Can result in garlic burns or blisters.

Touching the Penis

- Telugu People of South India touch the penis of the child to show respect.

===*FAST FACTS in a NUTSHELL*

> **Question:** The nurse notices bruises on the wrists and ankles of an infant. What intervention should be taken first?
>
> **Answer:** Complete a cultural assessment. Mongolian spots can be mistaken for bruises and can be located in atypical areas of the body.

CONCLUSION

Child abuse is not always obvious. The nurse is charged with the responsibility to know the warning signs of abuse and advocate for children accordingly. The reporting process does not require proof but simply all reasonable cause to suspect neglect or abuse. It only takes one phone call to the National Childline Reporting Center (available 24 hours at 1-800-422-4453) to initiate the process.

Early identification of abuse may result in early intervention and appropriate treatment for the child and the abuser.

REFERENCES AND FURTHER READING

Smith, M., & Segal, J. (2013, May). Child abuse and neglect: Recognizing, preventing, and reporting child abuse. *HelpGuide. org.* Retrieved from http://www.helpguide.org/mental/child_ abuse_physical_emotional_sexual_neglect.htm

U.S. Department of Health and Human Services & Administra-tion for Children and Families, Children's Bureau. (2011, December). *The child abuse prevention and treatment act (CAPTA) 2010.* Retrieved from http://www.acf.hhs.gov/programs/cb/resource/ capta2010

U.S. Department of Health and Human Services & Administra-tion for Children and Families. (n.d.). *Child Welfare Information Gateway: Spotlight on state child abuse reporting numbers.* Retrieved from http://www.childwelfare.gov/organizations/index.cfm

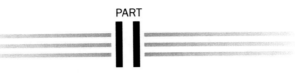

PART

II

Role of the Pediatric Nurse

7

Health Care Delivery in Pediatrics

Pediatric health care services are offered in a variety of settings including hospitals, public health department clinics, home care agencies, pediatrician offices, schools, and outpatient clinics. Each setting delivers specific pediatric-focused care by health care providers. The majority of children have health care coverage through their families' employer-sponsored health insurance coverage or through state-sponsored or subsidized programs.

This chapter reviews:

1. Sites and services for pediatric health care
2. Nursing role at pediatric health care sites

ROLE OF THE PEDIATRIC NURSE

Pediatric nurses provide care to infants, children, adolescents, and young adults, combining their nursing knowledge with detailed knowledge of growth and development to provide holistic care to their clients and families. The pediatric nurse plays an important role in the lives of his or her clients, both sick and healthy. The role of the pediatric nurse continues to evolve. Much of the role takes place in the community, as the population of pediatric patients in acute care has significantly declined, primarily due to the availability of immunizations.

ACUTE CARE SETTING

Hospital

Many hospitals designate a specific unit for the care of the pediatric population and include pediatric nurses with advanced knowledge in pediatrics. Hospital-sponsored pediatric education programs, pediatric-specific orientation, and professional pediatric certifications such as Pediatric Advanced Life Support (PALS) are required before assuming full duties on the pediatric unit.

Services provided include assessment and evaluation of the pediatric client with implementation of physician orders guiding care. Nursing techniques are frequently similar to those used when caring for adult clients but must include age-specific communication skills and size-specific equipment.

Hospitals also designate outpatient services to care for pediatric patients in specific areas such as diabetes, autism spectrum disorders, mental health, or rehabilitation services. Services provided assist the client and family in management, education, and follow-up necessary for a healthy lifestyle. A thorough knowledge of the community demographics and family support are essential.

FAST FACTS in a NUTSHELL

The PALS program was created as a joint effort between the American Heart Association (AHA) and the American Academy of Pediatrics (AAP) to assist professional health care providers in providing assessment and care to pediatric clients. The program was designed to help health care professionals streamline the treatment of pediatric patients and to ensure providers have the special training required to deal with injuries in children and infants who require advanced clinical care.

Pediatrician's Office

Provides specialized medical care by a physician(s) with advanced training in pediatrics. The total client population is pediatric clients from neonate through adolescents and, many times, the college years. The office environment is tailored to the interests and needs of children and includes various sizes of age-specific equipment. Services provided include triage of client symptoms, instruction in disease processes, symptom management, and anticipatory guidance to clients and their families.

Public Health Department

The public health department operates clinics throughout each state and provides research and statistics on a variety of health care trends. Although specifics may vary from state to state, the public health department provides free or reduced-cost screenings (physical, oral, hearing, vision) and immunizations. Services provided include public education on various health topics, monitoring of communicable diseases, preventive and primary care to diverse populations, and case management.

Home Care Agency

Home care agencies provide essential services to pediatric clients with health care needs, as well as support for the family within their home setting. With the understanding that it is best to maintain the child with the family at home, pediatric nurses bring nursing care and judgment to the home. Services provided include nursing assessment and identification of the needs of the family, health promotion and anticipatory guidance, promoting independence of the client and family, and linking the family to appropriate community resources.

Schools

Schools employ nurses to oversee school health policies and programs. The school nurse uses clinical knowledge and judgment to provide health care, perform screenings, and coordinate referrals. Services provided include serving as a liaison between school personnel, the client/family, the community, and the health care provider.

FAST FACTS in a NUTSHELL

The National Association of School Nurses (2014) recommends nurse-to-student ratios should be 1 to 750 for general populations, 1 to 225 in mainstreamed populations, and 1 to 125 in severely handicapped populations.

REFERENCES AND FURTHER READING

Hockenberry, M., & Wilson, D. (2013). *Wong's essentials of pediatric nursing* (9th ed.). St. Louis, MO: Elsevier.

Kyle, T., & Carman, S. (2013). *Essentials of pediatric nursing* (2nd ed.). Philadelphia, PA: Wolters Kluwer.

Leifer, G. (2011). *Introduction to maternity & pediatric nursing* (6th ed.). St. Louis, MO: Elsevier.

National Association of School Nurses. (2014, June). Retrieved from http://www.nasn.org

8

Hospitalization

Children are brought to the hospital for various reasons, which include:

- *An acute event leading to the immediate need of medical care*
- *A prolonged illness that has been exacerbated, leaving the hospital as the only agency available to provide evening or weekend care*
- *Utilization of the hospital as the only source of medical care*
- *Outpatient procedures*

Parents and children experience stress when a child is ill. Nursing communication is essential to update the child and family as information becomes available. When possible, it is essential to keep the parent and child together.

This chapter reviews:

1. Reasons for hospitalization
2. Children's reactions and behaviors related to hospitalization
3. Family considerations when a child is hospitalized

> Calmness is catching! Nurses who remain calm and confident in the care being provided filter that calmness to the parent and then to the pediatric client. Children feel stress from adults and become fearful and stressed themselves.

PREPARING THE CHILD FOR HOSPITALIZATION

When the opportunity presents, it is most beneficial for the child to be prepared for hospitalization to reduce anxiety and to help the child cope with the treatment regimen. Allowing the child to ask questions and verbalize fears enables the nurse to address the client's concerns, which may be real or fantasy. Honest answers promote trust.

When preparing a child for hospitalization, the nurse should:

- Provide a tour of the pediatric unit/room; stress similarity to home.
- Prepare the child according to age and developmental level.
- Be honest; the truth is less frightening.
- Be calm and unhurried; establish a relationship.
- Position self at the level of the client; speak at eye level.
- Provide information in a matter-of-fact manner; remain professional.
- Utilize books with pictures, dolls, or pamphlets that are age appropriate.
- Use simple, nonmedical words to promote client understanding.
- Stress that hospitalization is temporary; staff is working to make the client feel better so he or she can go home.
- Allow the child to pack his or her own belongings, if able.

ISSUES RELATED TO HOSPITALIZATION
PARENT/FAMILY

The nurse has the ability to make the hospital experience a positive one. When the child is hospitalized, the entire family is affected. Parents have fear and guilt related to their child's hospitalization—fear that the child will suffer or will spread the illness to others and fear that the child will transfer affection to the health care provider. It is the responsibility of the nurse to clarify misconceptions regarding the child's hospitalization and illness and to encourage confidence in the parents' ability to care for their child. The parent also has concerns about staying with the child at the hospital versus working or caring for other children. Depending upon the circumstance, it may be necessary for the parent to have a family member stay with the child or the child remain in the care of the nursing staff. Finances may also be impacted, as there may be eating, parking, and additional child-care expenses directly related to the hospitalization of the child. Also, siblings may be jealous of the parent's time spent with the hospitalized child or jealous of the attention that the hospitalized child is receiving.

FAST FACTS in a NUTSHELL

Though the health of the pediatric client is the main concern, it is also important to recognize the impact of the child's illness on the family and care for the family as well. Kind gestures such as offering a cup of coffee in the morning, sitting with the child while the parent showers, or providing an extra blanket during the night are comforting to the parent. Caring for the parent and family members strengthens their ability to care for their child.

PEDIATRIC CLIENT

The impact of hospitalization depends on the type of illness and the developmental level of the client. For a client with a first hospitalization, the client may be fearful of nursing interventions and the hospital environment. For the child who has had previous hospitalizations, the child has memories that provide either a comfort level or additional anxiety. It is important to understand a child's past experience, home life with sense of security, and amount of preparation given to the client before hospitalization.

The child's bed/room should be considered a safe area where no invasive procedures are completed. The child is able to rest and not be afraid that he or she will be surprised with painful procedures.

CONSIDERATIONS OF HOSPITALIZATION RELATED TO AGE

Infant

The nurse must utilize keen assessment skills to determine objective data in the infant. The child between 6 and 18 months of age may experience separation anxiety. Separation anxiety may be intense for both the child and parent. It often manifests as screaming and clinging to parents in the protest stage, depression and withdrawal or regression in the despair phase, or forming new relationships apart from the parents in the detachment phase.

Nursing Interventions

- Support parents who may be fatigued from consistently caring for an ill child.
- Place infants close to the nurses' station.
- Provide consistency with nurses interacting with an infant.

Toddler

The limited ability of toddlers to understand illness and follow directions, coupled with a "mind of their own," proves a challenge to nurses. Coaxing the toddler to cooperate with assessment techniques takes time and parental assistance. The toddler requires maximum contact with the parent, if possible. The toddler also experiences separation anxiety with intense reactions, increasing the difficulty in obtaining cooperation. Elicit parental assistance to the fullest of the parent's ability. If the parent appears to be frustrated or not able to tolerate a procedure, allow the parent to leave and have another nurse assist.

Nursing Interventions

- Offer choices to the toddler as appropriate.
- Allow the toddler to remain with the parent as the toddler is very fearful of separation.
- Encourage the parents to participate in their child's care.
- Provide consistency with nurses interacting with the toddler.
- Encourage comfort toys from home; a toddler is very possessive of belongings.

Preschool Age

The preschool client has some ability to provide subjective data and to assist with the completion of objective data. The preschooler has an increased understanding of illness and can be better prepared for procedures. The nurse must understand that the client utilizes magical thinking; thus, choosing words carefully to describe the disease process or nursing interventions is important. Preschoolers also may view care as a punishment. Though having had time away from parents to attend daycare or preschool, the client may still have periods of separation anxiety and want contact with the parent, especially when ill or scared.

Nursing Interventions

- Greet the child and allow the handling of equipment.
- Give choices when appropriate.
- Allow the child to play with toys or draw to express feelings.
- Explain procedures in clear, simple terms, free of medical jargon; no details.
- Allow the preschooler to participate in care as much as possible.
- Allow comfort toys from home or the opportunity to go to the playroom, if able.
- Encourage age-appropriate videos to pass time.

School Age

School-age children have the cognitive ability to understand and describe their illness. The client has the ability to note differences between normal and abnormal and cause and effect. The school-age client may cover up pain and symptoms to get home quicker.

This age group appreciates control in life and dislikes a loss of control. Truthfulness is important to maintain trust between the client and nurse. The school-age client may look admiringly at the nurse and be interested in the equipment used in medical care. Body image and modesty are also important; thus, the client can be embarrassed by components of a physical assessment. Although the school-age child wants the parent to be present when he or she is ill, separation from peers and school activities is also a concern.

Nursing Interventions

- Provide honesty in all interactions.
- Explain nursing interventions before they are completed.
- Encourage the expression of feelings.
- Maintain a routine schedule and allow contact with peers.
- Allow the child to go to the play room, if able.
- Place in a room with a child of the same age.

Adolescent

The adolescent has an adult's understanding of illness and can provide subjective data, answering questions with some detail. The adolescent attempts to maintain composure and control when ill. Body image is important to the adolescent and peers/school play a significant role in their life. Current technology allows clients to be hospitalized and remain in close contact with their peers. The adolescent may not follow the treatment regimen due to embarrassment, peer influence, and the work of maintaining the treatment regimen.

Nursing Interventions

- Encourage the adolescent to participate in care and make decisions when appropriate.
- Provide honesty in all interactions.
- Try to maintain a routine schedule and allow contact with peers.
- Offer books or movies to pass time.
- Encourage communication of thoughts and feelings.

NURSING CONSIDERATIONS RELATED TO HOSPITALIZATION

There are standards of care to be applied when caring for a client and his or her family. These standards are used as a guide. Most importantly, the nurse must remain flexible and try different approaches to interacting with the client and family.

- Greet the child and family by name and introduce yourself.
- When the pediatric client and family are admitted to the hospital, there is uncertainty about the regimen. Much client- and family-focused education is needed.
- Anticipate regressive behavioral changes such as incontinence or clinging. Educate parents that the behavioral changes are temporary.
- Relate all nursing interventions to the developmental level of the child. Encourage age-related activities and normal routines, when possible.
- Incorporate age-appropriate play into the daily regimen. Allow children to investigate nursing equipment with dolls.
- Keep the client room as a safe place. The client must rest and relax to heal.
- Provide an aesthetically pleasing, pediatric-friendly environment.

REFERENCES AND FURTHER READING

Hockenberry, M., & Wilson, D. (2013). *Wong's essentials of pediatric nursing* (9th ed.). St. Louis, MO: Elsevier.

Leifer, G. (2011). *Introduction to maternity & pediatric nursing* (6th ed.). St. Louis, MO: Elsevier.

9

Medication Administration and Special Procedures

It is not surprising that medical and nursing procedures/ interventions need adaptation to the pediatric population. Nurses cannot expect pediatric clients to tolerate or respond to medical procedures in the same manner as adults. Specially sized pediatric equipment is utilized to obtain specimens and provide medical care. Nurses must consider the age, developmental level, size (height/weight), and diagnosis of the client when providing appropriate care. This chapter outlines the differences in the care of the pediatric population and the nursing considerations.

This chapter reviews:

1. Pediatric medication administration and dosage calculations
2. Special procedures for the pediatric population
3. Pediatric procedure adaptation and pediatric sized equipment

ADJUSTING TO PEDIATRIC-SIZED CLIENTS

- Pediatric dosages are based on age recommendations, body weight (typically converted to kilograms), and body surface area (BSA) via a nomogram.

- While nurses administer medications per the physician's order, the nurse is responsible for ensuring that the medication is within the client's safe-dose range.
- Notify the physician if medication dosage is outside of the safe-dose range.
- Double check high-risk and regulated medications with a second nurse.
- Perform the six rights of medication administration. Engage parental assistance if needed in administering the medication.
- The growth and maturation of each organ system affects the metabolism and excretion of medication.

PEDIATRIC SAFE-DOSE CALCULATIONS

- If the dosage is determined according to age, compare the age of the client with dosage guidelines.
- If the dosage is determined by body surface area, obtain height and weight to determine the total area of the skin.
- If the dosage is determined by weight, a mathematical calculation is required.

The nurse must ensure a safe dose and proper medication administration for the pediatric client. Calculating a pediatric dosage depends on determining the milligram (mg) of medication per kilogram (kg) of weight.

1. Calculating kilograms of weight is determined by:

$$\frac{\text{Weight in pounds}}{2.2\,\text{kilograms}} = \text{Weight in kilograms}$$

2. Once the weight in kilograms is determined, multiply by the dosage per kilogram of weight. Pay particular attention to the "per day" or "per dose" calculation needed.

DOSAGE CALCULATION

The nurse must be able to perform a variety of dosage calculations to determine accurate amounts (tablets, milliliters, or milligrams) according to weight. Various calculation formulas determine the accurate dose. Consult a drug calculation book for the formulas and practice problems of ratio/proportion, dimensional analysis, and alternate formula of the desired dose divided by the known amount multiplied by the quantity of medication.

Dosage Calculation Examples

The client is ordered Ativan 3 mg IM h.s. Ativan is supplied in a prefilled dosage syringe of 4 mg/mL. How many milliliters will the nurse administer?

1. **Ratio/proportion**: This method requires that the known proportion and the unknown proportion be set in the same format.

   Thus: 4 mg:1 mL :: 3 mg: xmL

   Divide both sides by 4 mg =

   $$\frac{4\,mg x mL}{4\,mg/mL} = \frac{3\,mg/mL}{4\,mg/mL} = x = 3/4 \text{ or } 0.75 \text{ mL}$$

2. **Dimensional analysis**: This method requires that the unknown be kept on the left side of the equation.

   $$\text{Thus,} x mL = \frac{mL}{4\,mg} \times \frac{3\,mg}{x} = \frac{3}{4} = 0.75\,mL$$

3. **Alternate formula**: This method can be used if the physician's order is in one system of measurement.

   The formula is $\dfrac{\text{Desired}}{\text{Available}} \times \text{Quantity}$

   $$\frac{3\,mg\,(\text{Desired})}{4\,mg\,(\text{Available})} \times 1\,mL\,(\text{Quantity}) = \frac{3}{4} = 0.75\,mL$$

════════════════════════ *FAST FACTS in a NUTSHELL*

The most common mathematical error when calculating medication dosage is in the placement of the decimal point. An inaccurate placement can increase a dosage tenfold.

MEDICATION ADMINISTRATION

Pediatric medication administration shares many nursing standards with adult medication administration. The first standard is the six rights of medication administration. Even though the six rights do not incorporate the age of the child, it ensures accuracy through the use of:

- The right drug
- The right dose
- The right time
- The right patient
- The right route
- The right documentation

Considering the standard of atraumatic pediatric care, physicians order medications to be administered via the least invasive route to minimize client trauma. Routes of medication administration vary according to age and diagnosis. Education according to the developmental level is important for children; that is, "what" the medication is and "why" it is being given.

Oral Medications

The oral route is the route of choice, providing the options of liquid medication administered by a syringe for infants and tablets/pills for children, who are able to swallow solids. Prior to any medication administration, the nurse must determine that the dosage is safe. Once completed, the nurse administers medications using the following technique:

- Infants/toddlers:
  - Draw up liquid in an oral syringe, inject along the side of the mouth in small amounts to prevent aspiration. It may be necessary to have another person/parent stabilize the infant's hands or head.
  - Having the client pucker the lips similar to forming a kiss face elongates the canal, requiring the infant to swallow the medication rather than spitting it out.
  - A nipple may be used to allow the child to suck the medication.

Never give oral medications to a crying child due to the risk of aspiration.

- Preschool/school-age children:
  - May be able to hold a medicine cup (30 cc) and drink the liquid from the cup.
  - Inquire if the child can safely chew or swallow a whole tablet or pill prior to pill administration.
  - If the medication is unpleasant, the child may suck on something frozen to dull the taste or the nurse can mix the mediation in a small amount of sweet liquid.
  - If the child wishes, have the child pinch his or her nose during medication administration.
- Adolescents:
  - Medication administration is per adult techniques.
  - The adolescent is typically cooperative in administering medications, as oral medications do not cause discomfort.
  - The nurse may hand the medication to the adolescent and observe the adolescent ingesting it.

Ophthalmic Medications

Assistance is best when administering ophthalmic medications to a pediatric client. Assist the client into a supine or sitting position. The infant/toddler may move or reach for the nurse when the nurse is preparing to administer the drop. Also, the pediatric client may squint, blink frequently, or be apprehensive to have medication placed in the eye.

- Infants/toddlers/preschoolers/school-age/adolescents:
  - Tilt the client's head back, gently press the skin under the lower eyelid, and pull the lower lid away slightly until a small pouch is visible.
  - Ask the client to look up.
  - Insert the ointment or drop (one at a time) and close the eye for a few minutes to keep the medicine in the eye.
  - Apply light pressure to the lacrimal punctum for 1 minute to prevent an unpleasant taste

Otic Medications

Otic medications are typically well tolerated by all age groups. It is important to ensure that the medication warms to room temperature prior to administration. Massage the outer area of the ear for a couple of minutes following medication administration. Assistance is best when administering to infants/toddlers as they cannot follow the instructions for positioning.

- Infants/toddlers/preschoolers/school-age/adolescents:
- Shake otic suspensions well before administration.
- For children less than 3 years, pull the outer ear outward and downward before instilling drops. For children 3 years or older, pull the outer ear outward and upward.
- Keep child on side for 2 minutes and instill a cotton plug into the ear.

Nasal Medications

Nasal instillation of fluid may be for medication administration or upper respiratory irrigation to remove crusted drainage. Infants, toddlers, and preschoolers resist liquids administered to the upper airway. Assistance in administration is best. A football hold may be used for infants. Education to school-age children and adolescents promotes an understanding of the procedure and cooperation.

- Infants/toddlers/preschoolers/school-age/adolescents:
  - Clear the nose of secretions prior to administration. A nasal aspirator (bulb syringe) or a cotton swab may be used in infants and young children. Ask older children to blow their nose.
  - Tilt the child's head back over a pillow and squeeze the dropper without touching the nostril.
  - Keep child's head tilted back for 2 minutes.

Suppositories

Suppositories are frequently administered when the pediatric client cannot tolerate oral administration. Infants typically tolerate the procedure well, as they are used to having their diaper changed and contact with the anal region for hygiene. Toddlers and preschoolers are most resistant, often bearing down to remove the suppository administered. Embarrassment is common in school-age or adolescent clients.

- Infants/toddlers/preschoolers/school-age/adolescents:
  - Keep refrigerated for easier administration.
  - Wearing gloves, moisten the rounded end with water or petroleum jelly prior to insertion.
  - Use your pinky finger for children less than 3 years old and your index finger for those 3 years or older.
  - Insert the suppository into the rectum about 1/2 to 1 inch beyond the sphincter.
  - If the suppository slides out, insert it a little farther than before. Hold the buttocks together for a few minutes.
  - Have the client hold the position for 20 minutes, if possible.

Topical Medications

Topical ointments/lotions may be administered to provide analgesia prior to an invasive procedure, decrease a sensation such as pruritus, or contain medication for systemic absorption. Topical medications are generally tolerated well by all ages.

- Infants/toddlers/preschoolers/school-age/adolescents:
  - Clean affected area and dry well prior to application.
  - Apply a thin layer to the skin and rub in gently.
  - Do not apply coverings over the area unless instructed to do so by the prescriber.

Nebulizers and Metered-Dose Inhalers

Nebulizers and metered-dose inhalers deliver medications in aerosol form through the lower respiratory tract. Infants/toddlers/school-age clients need assistance via a specially sized mask to ensure an appropriate snug fit and obtain the medication. Spacers are used for metered-dose inhalers, holding the medication in the chamber until the client draws the medication down the respiratory tract. Parents are also helpful to encourage cooperation in all age groups and ensure deep breathing to instill the medication deep into the respiratory tract.

- Infants/toddlers/preschoolers/school-age/adolescents:
  - Obtain specially sized equipment with medication.

- Allow the child to assist as much as possible.
- Provide distraction or gaming during nebulizer treatment to pass the time.
- Encourage deep breathing.

Injectable Medications

Injectable medications cause anxiety and typically discomfort to all age groups. Education in age-appropriate terms is needed immediately before the procedure to prepare and elicit assistance. The nurse should never lie to the client or minimize the client's feelings of anxiety. Parents provide a sense of comfort for the client and should be encouraged to stay during the procedure, if possible. Restraint may be needed in any age group to decrease the movement of the needle while injecting.

Encourage age-appropriate comfort measures and distractions, such as:

- Have the parent at the client's head talking and touching the client to provide comfort.
- Offer sucrose pacifiers for infants.
- Distract the client during site preparation.
- Have the parent hold the client's hand during the injection.
- Instruct the client that he or she can cry or squeeze someone's hand but cannot move.
- Immediately following the injection, allow the parent to soothe the child.
- Offer play therapy as a distraction or to decrease anxiety.
- Perform in a treatment room, away from safe area.

FAST FACTS in a NUTSHELL

When considering injection sites for medication administration, consider the following:

- Age and size of client
- Medication amount, viscosity, and type of medication
- Muscle mass, client use of muscle, accessibility of site
- Treatment and number of injections

Use the smallest-gauge of needle possible.

| Nursing Consideration: | May apply a topical analgesic, typically containing lidocaine, to the site 60 minutes prior to the injection. |

Intradermal
- Administer in the inner surface of the forearm
- Use a tuberculin (TB) syringe with a 26- to 30-gauge needle
- Insert at a 15-degree angle with the bevel up
- Inject directly; do not aspirate or massage

Subcutaneous
- Commonly given in the subcutaneous tissue of the lateral aspect of the upper arm, abdomen, and anterior thigh
- Inject no more than 0.5 mL of fluid
- Use a 1 mL syringe with a 26- to 30-gauge needle
- Insert at a 45-degree angle for children with less muscle mass or a 90-degree angle for children with adequate muscle mass

Intramuscular
- Use a 22- to 25-gauge 1/2- to 1-inch needle
- Procedure depends on muscle site
  - Vastus lateralis: Recommended for infants and small children.
    Patient position supine, side-lying, or sitting.
    Inject up to 0.5 mL for infants.
    Inject up to 2 mL for children.
  - Ventrogluteal:
    Patient position supine, side-lying, or prone.
    Inject up to 0.5 mL for infants.
    Inject up to 2 mL for children.
  - Deltoid: Recommended for children and adults, if appropriate. Position the child sitting, preferably with the parent for young children, or also can be standing.
    Inject up to 1 mL.

FAST FACTS in a NUTSHELL

To ensure the most pain-free of injections, consider changing the needle after puncturing a stopper.

Intravenous Medications

It may be necessary for the pediatric client to require intravenous (IV) support via IV solutions and/or medications. This procedure causes discomfort and anxiety in all age groups. Age-appropriate communication is given immediately before the procedure so that anxiety does not build. Similar age-appropriate comfort measures and support, as given with injection therapy, are utilized.

Peripheral IV Catheter

May assess multiple sites:

Infants:
- Scalp
- Hand/forearm
- Foot

Toddlers:
- Scalp
- Hand/forearm

Preschoolers/School-Age/Adolescents:

- Hand/forearm (choose nondominant hand if possible)

- Prepare all equipment, including priming of tubing, prior to entering room.
- Catheter size depends on the size of vein. Use a 24 gauge or butterfly for neonates and small infants. Otherwise, use a 20- to 22-gauge catheter.
- Spend time determining "best" vein for use. This may limit multiple venipunctures.
- Use a transilluminator to locate vein.
- Use topical analgesic; administer 60 minutes prior to procedure, if able.
- Secure firmly; attach extension tubing to decrease movement.
- Wrap with a stretchy material.

Central IV Catheter

Nontunneled
- Peripherally inserted central catheter for short-term therapy (PICC line)

Tunneled
- Long-term catheter or implanted infusion port

- Inserted by individuals (RN or MD) with special training.
- Assist with procedure, providing support to the RN/MD and the client.

Fluid intoxication can occur during IV fluid replacement. Infants are especially vulnerable to fluid volume excess. To determine the daily fluid maintenance requirements, use the following formula:

Body Weight (kg)	Amount of Fluid per Day
1–10 kg	100 mL/kg
11–20 kg	1,000 mL (total above) plus 50 mL/kg for each kg above 10 kg
Above 20 kg	1,500 mL (i.e., total of above two steps) plus 20 mL/kg >20

NURSING PROCEDURES FOR THE PEDIATRIC POPULATION

Nurses need to be skilled at various nursing procedures for the pediatric population. Following are the most common pediatric nursing procedures. As always, consult your institution's policy and procedure manual for specific care considerations.

Enema Administration

Enema administration can be uncomfortable. Look for clues that cramping may be occurring and stop or slow administration. If administering multiple enemas, monitor for signs of electrolyte imbalance.

- Gather all supplies (enema bag, lubricant, enema solution as ordered); wash hands/glove.
- Explain procedure in age-appropriate terms.
- Position client:
  - Infant/toddler: On abdomen with knees bent
  - Child/adolescent: On left side with right leg flexed toward chest

- Remove cap, lubricate tip, insert into rectum:
  - Infant: Insert 2.5 to 4 cm (1–1.5 inch)
  - Child: Insert 5 to 7.5 cm (2–3 inches)
- Unclamp tubing, administer prescribed volume.

- Guidelines:
- Infants: 250 mL or less
- Toddler/preschooler: 250 to 500 mL
- School-age: 500 to 1,000 mL
- Adolescent: 1,500 to 2,000 mL (adult amount)

Obtaining a Urine Culture/Specimen Using a Urine Bag

Used for infants and small children who are not yet toilet trained.

- Cleanse perineal area well and pat dry.
- Apply urine bag (some facilities use benzoin to aid with bag adhesion).
  - For boys: Place bag around the penis and, depending upon size, a portion of the testes may be inside the bag as well.
  - For girls: Apply the narrow portion of the bag on the perineal space between the anal and vulvar area first then spread out the remaining section.
- Tuck the bag downward inside the diaper, maintaining the upright position of the bag to discourage leakage.
- Check frequently.
- When urine is present in bag, hold bag vertically, pinching off the top portion while gently pulling bag from skin.
- Place bag with urine inside into cup for transport to lab.

Nasal Suctioning Using a Bulb Syringe

Recall that infants are obligatory nose breathers. Also, cough reflexes are not fully developed in infants, collecting mucus in the throat. To assist with maintaining an open airway during periods of upper airway congestion, a bulb syringe is used to withdraw nasal secretions. Infants protest the use of a bulb syringe by crying and turning their heads away. Assistance is needed to stabilize the head.

- Wash hands.
- Hold the tip of the bulb between the middle finger and fore-finger. The bulb should touch the palm of the hand.

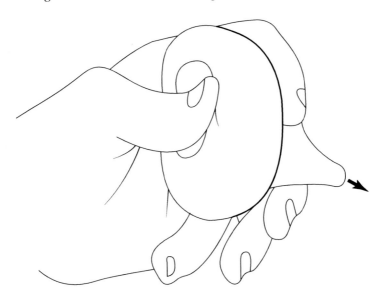

- Before inserting the tip into the nose, use the thumb to push out the air.
- Insert the tip of the bulb into either the mouth or the nose and slowly release. Suction is created as the thumb releases pressure on the bulb. This will create suction and remove mucus or fluid from the infant's mouth or nose.
- If the bulb does not reinflate, the tip is against the cheek or lining of the nose or is blocked by thick mucus. If pulling back on the bulb does not reinflate the bulb, remove and clean the bulb syringe.
- Remove the bulb syringe from the mouth or nose. Use the thumb to push mucus or fluids out of the bulb syringe onto a tissue or paper towel.
- Clean the bulb syringe with tap water between suction attempts.
- Repeat as needed. Allow the infant to recover and breathe between each suction attempt.
- Let the bulb syringe air dry.

REFERENCES AND FURTHER READING

Hockenberry, M., & Wilson, D. (2013). *Wong's essentials of pediatric nursing* (9th ed.). St. Louis, MO: Elsevier.

Leifer, G. (2011). *Introduction to maternity & pediatric nursing* (6th ed.). St. Louis, MO: Elsevier.

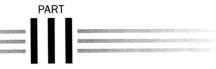

PART

III

System Review of Common Pediatric Disorders

10

Emotional or Behavioral Disorders

Early childhood experiences and situations that disrupt the family can have a lasting impact on the child and on personality formation. Being raised in a dysfunctional family may also lead to a failure to develop a sense of trust, excess fears, misdirected anger, low-self-esteem, lack of confidence, and/or feelings of loss of control over self or the environment. A child who is dealing with feelings of guilt and blame will struggle in an attempt to cope and deal with the stress of daily life. Often, these struggles result in behavioral disorders.

This chapter reviews:

1. Common emotional and behavioral disorders found in children
2. Childhood eating disorders
3. Common substances abused by children and adolescents
4. Warning signs of suicide ideation in adolescents

EMOTIONAL OR BEHAVIORAL DISORDERS

The disorders included in this category, when left untreated, can interfere with the child's total functioning. Although no exact cause is proven, some behavioral disorders are linked to genetic origin or a defect in neurogenesis in the early weeks of fetal life. Some are associated with self-perception, increased problems in scholastic competence, social acceptance, or behavioral conduct in children. Children with emotional or behavioral disorders are at higher risk for developing maladaptive behavior patterns that hinder psychosocial adjustment, precipitate anxiety, and interfere with self-concept and mood.

Autism—Autism Spectrum Disorder (ASD)

Description

- A developmental disorder that involves impaired social interaction, communication, and interests
- Occurs in 6.69 per 1,000 children
- More common in males

Manifestations

- Motor–sensory, cognitive, and behavioral dysfunctions
- No smile or joyful expression by 6 months or thereafter
- No back-and-forth sharing of sounds, smiles, or other facial expressions by 9 months
- No babbling by 12 months
- No pointing, showing, reaching, or waving by 12 months
- No words by 16 months
- No meaningful two-word phrases by 24 months
- Any loss of speech, babbling, or social skills at any age
- Failure to make eye contact and look at others
- Poor attention behavior or poor orientation to name
- Lack of interest in engaging in play with other children (Autism Speaks, n.d.)

Diagnostic Criteria

- Modified checklist for autism in toddlers—revised M-CHAT-R/F by Dr. Diana L. Robins
  - If the child fails the M-CHAT-R/F, further evaluation is indicated to assess for the diagnosis of autism spectrum disorder.
  - M-CHAT-R/F assessment tool and instructions for use are located in Appendix B

- *Diagnostic and Statistical Manual of Mental Disorders*, fifth edition (*DSM-5*)
  - The diagnosis is based on history and presentation of the manifestations.

Interventions

- Early identification and intervention by trained therapists
  - Depression, anxiety, hyperactivity, and obsessive–compulsive behaviors are sometimes an underlying behavior condition and may need to be treated
- Goal of therapy is to maximize the ability to live independently
- Provide well-structured home and school environments
- Behavioral training and management, positive reinforcement, and/or applied behavioral analysis (ABA)
- Occupational and physical therapies specific to identified deficiencies

Attention-Deficit/Hyperactivity Disorder (ADHD)

Description

- A developmentally inappropriate degree of gross motor activity, impulsivity, and inattention in the school or home setting that begins before age 7 years, lasts more than 6 months, and is not related to the existence of any other central nervous system illness
- Most common neurobehavioral disorder
- More common in boys
- Occurs more often in some families (genetic connection suggested)
- Other possible causes and risk factors include:
  - Brain injury
  - Environmental exposures (e.g., lead)
  - Alcohol and tobacco use during pregnancy
  - Premature delivery or low birth weight

Manifestations

- Inattention/ distractibility—at least three of the following:
  - Is easily distracted

- Needs calm atmosphere to work
- Fails to complete work
- Does not appear to listen
- Has difficulty concentrating without 1:1 instruction
- Needs information repeated
- Impulsivity—at least three of the following:
  - Disruptive with other children
  - Talks out in class, overly talkative
  - Extremely excitable
  - Cannot wait turn
  - Requires much supervision
- Hyperactivity—at least two of the following:
  - Climbs on furniture
  - Fidgets
  - Always "on the go"
  - Cannot stay seated
  - Does things in a loud/noisy way
- Learning disabilities often occur with ADHD associated with difficulties in listening, understanding, ability to express ideas, differentiating words that sound/look alike, remembering personal information, motor coordination, confusing left and right, difficulty concentrating, impatience, and dyslexia

Diagnostic Criteria

- No single test to diagnosis
- History of the behavior according to parent, teacher, and child
- Symptoms present in two or more settings (school, home, clubs)

Interventions

- Stimulant medications to boost and balance neurotransmitter levels in the brain. Examples include methylphenidate (Concerta, Metadate, Ritalin, others), dextroamphetamine (Dexedrine), dextroamphetamine-amphetamine (Adderall XR), and lisdexamfetamine (Vyvanse). Other medications used to treat ADHD include atomoxetine (Strattera) and antidepressants such as bupropion (Wellbutrin, others).
- Behavior therapy—Teachers and parents can learn behavior-changing strategies for dealing with difficult situations. These strategies may include token reward systems and timeouts.

- Psychotherapy—This allows older children with ADHD to talk about issues that bother them, explore negative behavioral patterns, and learn ways to deal with their symptoms.
- Parenting skills training—This can help parents develop ways to understand and guide their child's behavior.
- Family therapy—Family therapy can help parents and siblings deal with the stress of living with someone who has ADHD.
- Social skills training—This can help children learn appropriate social behavior.

Anorexia Nervosa

Description

- An eating disorder characterized by a refusal to maintain normal body weight and by severe weight loss in the absence of physical causes.
- The mean age of onset is 13.75 years; range is 10 to 25 years.
- Tend to be perfectionists, academic high achievers, conforming, and conscientious.

Manifestations

- Failure to maintain the minimum normal weight for age and height (less than 85% of expected weight)
- Distorted body image
- Intense fear of gaining weight; relentless pursuit of thinness
- Refusal to eat or highly restrictive eating
- Compulsive exercise
- Amenorrhea, hair loss with lanugo hair on back, face, and extremities
- Cold intolerance, low blood pressure, and diminishing socialization with peers

Diagnostic Criteria

- Based on detailed history of the child's behavior from parents and teachers
- Clinical observations of the child's behavior and psychological testing contribute to the diagnosis
- Weight relative to the average for age; consistently maintains a body weight 15% below average

Interventions

- A brief hospital/clinic admission may be required to correct electrolyte imbalances, restore nutrients, and stabilize weight.
- Anorexia is usually treated with a combination of individual therapy (usually including both cognitive and behavioral techniques), family therapy, nutritional rehabilitation, and behavior modification.
- Weekly eating disorder support groups for continued support.
  - Approximately 25% fully recover, 50% improve, 25% do poorly.

Bulimia

Description

- An eating disorder characterized by repeated episodes of binge eating followed by inappropriate compensatory behaviors, such as self-induced vomiting, fasting, or excessive exercise, and misuse of laxatives, diuretics, or other medications.
- More common in older adolescent girls and young women.

Manifestations

- Family dysfunctions are usually present
- Binge eating followed by purging to cope with feelings of guilt, depression, or low self-esteem
- As the disease progresses, loss of control over binge/purge cycle increases
- Muscle weakness and electrolyte imbalance with emetic and laxative use
- Hand lesions (Russell's sign) indicate repeated attempts to induce vomiting
- Erosion of teeth enamel
- Chronic esophagitis, sore throat, difficulty swallowing, and parotitis
- Esophageal tears, hiatal hernia, and/or spontaneous bleeding in the eye with severe vomiting

Most people with bulimia are within the normal weight range.

Diagnostic Criteria

- Based on history and physical exam and criteria from the American Psychiatric Association
- The criteria for a diagnosis of bulimia according to the *Diagnostic and Statistical Manual of Mental Disorders*, fifth edition (*DSM-5;* American Psychiatric Association, 2013) include:
  - Repeated episodes of binge eating, including eating an abnormally large amount of food and feeling a lack of control over eating
  - These behaviors occur at least twice a week for at least 3 months
  - Self-esteem is overly influenced by body shape and weight
  - The eating disorder behavior does not occur during periods of anorexia

Interventions

- Restore electrolyte imbalance (cardiac monitoring if indicated)
- Individual, group, and/or family psychotherapy
- Nutritional counseling and support groups

Childhood Obesity

Description

- When intake of food exceeds expenditure resulting in elevated body mass index (BMI) for age (see Manifestations)
- Related to a combination of heredity, diet, sedentary lifestyle, and social, cultural, and psychological factors
- Considered a family problem since parents and children share in the habits, lifestyle, and manifestations associated with the disorder

Manifestations

- BMI
  - BMI over 18 in children 5 to 9 years
  - BMI over 22 to 24 in children 13 to 17 years
- Altered eating habits (amounts, time of intake, types of food, and cues for eating)

Diagnostic Criteria

- Based on history, physical exam, and BMI

Interventions

- Education of parents, children, educators, health care providers, and general public
- Nutritional counseling for the family on portion control, healthy food choices, and exercise
- Family and individual behavior modification therapy

FAST FACTS in a NUTSHELL

Question: What is the most prevalent complication of childhood obesity?

Answer: Childhood obesity often leads to life-long obesity, placing adults at risk for medical complications that include hypertension, diabetes, coronary heart disease, stroke, and colorectal cancer.

Substance Abuse

Description

- The adopted use of nicotine, alcohol, or chemical substances as means of coping with feelings of depression, anxiety, restlessness, or chronic feelings of boredom or emptiness
- Can be a voluntary behavior or an involuntary/physiologic response (physical dependence)
- See Table 10.1 for list of commonly abused substances among children and adolescents

TABLE 10.1 Commonly Abused Substances

Name of Substance	Street Names	Effects
Tobacco/Nicotine/e-Cigarettes		Enhances concentration, memory, alertness, and arousal. Decreases anxiety
Alcohol	Booze, Hooch, Satan's Nectar	CNS depressant that sparks energy, elation, and excitement
Amphetamine/Biphetamine/Dexedrine	Bennies, Black Beauties, Crosses, Hearts, LA Turnaround, Speed, Truck Drivers, Uppers	Increased energy and alertness. Decreased appetite
Cocaine	Blizzard, Blow, C, Candy, Coke, Crack, Choreboy, Dust, Going Skiing, Nose Candy, Schoolboy, Snow, Toot	Intense rush, arousal, increased confidence
Coricidin (HBP)/DXM/Dextromethorphan	Skittles, Trip Cs, Robotrip	Sense of well-being, tripping
Fentanyl/Duragesic/Synthetic Opiate Analgesic	Fent, Apache, China Girl, China White, Dance Fever, Friend, Goodfella, Jackpot, Murder 8, TNT, Tango and Cash	High, euphoria, and relaxation
Flunitrazepam/Rohypnol	Date rape drug, Rope, Rib, Roofies	Powerful sedative
Formaldehyde/Embalming Fluid–Dipped Cigarettes or Joints	Amp, Wet, Fry, Illy, Dank, Water, Hydro	High like PCP
Gamma Hydroxybutyrate(GHB)	Grevious Bodily Harm, G, Georgia Home Boy, Liquid X, Cups	Euphoric high, aphrodisiac, hallucinations

(continued)

TABLE 10.1 Commonly Abused Substances (continued)

Name of Substance	Street Names	Effects
Heroin/Opiate	Cheese, China White, Diesel, Dope, H, Horse, Jet Fuel, Junk, Smack, Stamp (small bag), Sugar, Tar	Warmth and contentment
Inhalants: Solvents/Aerosols/Refrigerants	Bic lighter, White Out, glue, markers, hair spray, paint, WD40, body sprays, room deodorizers, can air, nail polish remover, cow manure, vomit, carbon dioxide cartridges, amyl nitrate, Rush, Bolt, Whippit, Jenkum	Mind altering, numbing
Ketamine Hydrochloride	K Hole, Special K, Vitamin K, Super K	Hallucination, altered perceptions, dissociations
Lysergic Acid Diethylamide (LSD)	Acid, Blotter, Windowpane	Psychedelic experience, colorful visual illusions
Marijuana/Cannabis	Mary Jane, Pot, Smoke, Weed Amp = cigar dipped in formaldehyde Blunt = cigar filled with marijuana Kreeper = cigar saturated in bug spray	Relaxed, happy, talkative, increased appetite
Synthetic Marijuana/Spice	K2, Fake Weed, Yucatan Fire, Skunk, Moon Rocks, Herbal Incense	Mind-altering effects

Methamphetamine	Ice, Crank, Meth, Crystal	CNS stimulant, euphoria and rush, decreased appetite
Methylenedioxymethamphetamine (MDMA)	Ecstasy, X, Love Drug, Molly	Euphoric rush, heightened sensation, hallucinations, increased energy, affectionate, decreased appetite
Methylphenidate/Ritalin	Kibbles & Bits, Pineapple	Amphetamine-like CNS stimulant, euphoria, wakefulness, alertness
Oxycontin/Percocet/Demeral	Oxy, OC, Oxy Cotton, Mrs. O, Percs, Biscuits	Euphoria, relaxation
Phencyclidine (PCP)	Angel Dust, Satan	Hallucinogen and dissociative drug
Psilocybin (4-phosphoryloxy-N, N-dimethyltryptamine)	Mushrooms, Magic Mushrooms, Shrooms	Hallucinations
Salvia Devinorum (herb in the mint family)	Shepherdess's Herb, Maria Pastora, Magic Mint, Sally-D	Hallucinations, multiple realities
Synthetic Cathinones/Bath Salts/ Khat Plant	Ivory Wave, Bloom, Cloud Nine, Lunar Wave, Vanilla Sky, White Lightning, Scarface	Amphetamine-like stimulant; increased euphoria and sex drive

CNS, central nervous system.

Manifestations

- Dependent on *patterns of drug use*
    - A markedly diminished effect with continued use of the same amount of substance results in greater desire/use of substance
- Dependent on *types of drugs abused*
    - Tobacco/nicotine
        - Irritable, frustrated, anxious, difficulty concentrating, depressed mood
    - Alcohol
        - Aggression, lethargy, impaired coordination, judgment, and perception
    - Chemical substances (prescription or street drugs)
        - Opiates: Constricted pupils, respiratory depression, euphoria, lethargy, coma
        - Depressants: Slurred speech, ataxia, hyperexcitability, impaired judgment, violent
        - Stimulants: Hypertension, tachycardia, personality change, hyperactive
        - Hallucinogens: Delayed response, hyperthermia, increased sensory awareness, confusion, hallucinations, paranoia, increased hunger
        - Inhalants: Sore throat, cough, runny nose, impaired perception, loss of consciousness

Diagnostic Criteria

- Significant impairment or distress as manifested by three or more of the following:
    - Need to increase amount to achieve desired effect
    - Withdrawal syndrome
    - Substance taken in larger amounts or over a longer period than intended
    - Unsuccessful efforts/desire to cut down on use
    - Increased time spent on thinking about, obtaining, using, or recovering from substance
    - Important social, work, or recreational activities are given up
    - Substance use is continued despite knowledge of physical or psychological problems

Interventions

- Safe management while removing the dependent chemicals in acute drug detoxification
- Rehabilitation may be required as inpatient, outpatient, or a combination of both
  - First step is to admit dependence on chemical(s) and a desire to make a change in behavior
  - Focus on relearning and adapting coping behaviors without using chemicals
  - Establishing a support system for remaining chemical free
- Individual counseling, group therapy, and 12-step self-help groups such as Alcoholics Anonymous and Narcotics Anonymous have provided assistance for many

A comprehensive website on drug abuse, with research and treatment reports, can be found at the National Institute on Drug Abuse at www.drugabuse.gov.

Suicide

Description

- Deliberate act of self-injury with the intent to result in death
- Suicidal ideation—thoughts about committing suicide
- Suicide attempt—unsuccessful attempt to cause injury or death

Manifestations

- Presence of an active psychiatric disorder (such as depression, bipolar disorder, substance abuse, conduct disorders)
- The expression/communication of thoughts of suicide, death, dying, or the afterlife (in a context of sadness, boredom, hopelessness, or negative feelings)
- Recent severe stressor (e.g., difficulties in dealing with sexual orientation, sexual abuse, unplanned pregnancy, significant real or anticipated loss, rejection of close friend, family discord or loss, humiliating experience, or legal issues)

Diagnostic Criteria

- Warning signs of suicide:
  - Preoccupation with death
  - Gives away cherished possessions
  - Exhibits loss of interest or energy
  - Noted change in sleep pattern
  - Physical complaints or repeated health care visits
  - Reckless or antisocial behavior
  - Sudden change in school grades
  - Distant, sad, flat affect
  - Describes self as worthless
  - Social withdrawal from friends, activities, or interests
  - Dramatic change in appetite
  - Sudden cheerfulness after deep depression

FAST FACTS in a NUTSHELL

Risk for successful suicide increases if the individual identifies the following:
- *Plan*—Is there a plan of action?
- *Means*—Is there a means to carry out the plan?
- *Absence of resources*—Is there someone who can help?

Interventions

- Active depression or suicide ideation needs inpatient care to ensure safety.
- If risk for suicide is identified, the nurse needs to:
  - Show interest and support
  - Ask if he/she is thinking about suicide
  - Be direct; talk openly and freely about suicide
  - Be willing to listen; allow for expression of feelings; accept the feelings
  - Be nonjudgmental and don't lecture on the value of life
  - Don't give advice or ask "why"; this encourages defensiveness
  - Offer empathy, not sympathy
  - Don't be sworn to secrecy; seek support

- Offer hope that alternatives are available
- Take action! Remove means! Get help from individuals or agencies specializing in crisis intervention and suicide prevention

CONCLUSION

A knowledgeable, caring, and supportive nature is valuable when caring for a child with emotional or behavioral disorders. Approaching the child and family with a caring, nonjudgmental attitude is the key.

Emotional or behavioral disorders place children at higher risk for developing maladaptive behavior patterns that hinder psychosocial adjustment, precipitate anxiety, and interfere with self-concept and mood. As a nurse, you need to know that treatment plans require the coordination of a multidisciplinary team.

REFERENCES AND FURTHER READING

American Psychiatric Association. (2013). *Diagnostic and statistical manual of mental disorders* (5th ed.). Arlington, VA: Author.

Autism Speaks. (n.d.). *What is autism?* Retrieved from http://www.autismspeaks.org

Hockenberry, M., & Wilson, D. (2013). *Wong's essentials of pediatric nursing* (9th ed.). St. Louis, MO: Elsevier.

Leifer, G. (2011). *Introduction to maternity & pediatric nursing* (6th ed.). St. Louis, MO: Elsevier.

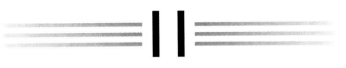

Neurologic and Chromosomal Disorders

The neurologic system is composed of the body's nervous system. Neurologic disorders are classified according to primary location affected, type of dysfunction, or cause. The nervous system is the body's communication center; it receives and transmits messages to all parts of the body. Our nervous system is also essential in memory and learning. Many neurologic abnormalities are a result of congenital malformations and/or chromosomal errors (birth defects). After reviewing this chapter, you will have a basic understanding of the most common neurological or chromosomal disorders found in children.

This chapter reviews:

1. Pathophysiology of the neurologic system in pediatric clients
2. Nursing care required for pediatric clients with various neurologic conditions
3. Instruction necessary for families of clients with neurologic conditions

VARIATIONS IN PEDIATRIC ANATOMY AND PHYSIOLOGY

The structures of the nervous system (neural tube development) occur during the third to fourth week of fetal life. This structure eventually becomes the CNS. A child is born with two fontanelles (the anterior closes at approximately 2 years of age; the posterior closes at approximately 2 to 3 months of age) to allow for molding during the birth process and allow for increases in intracranial pressure or brain growth. Increased brain growth and specialization of function occur most rapidly from birth to 4 years old. Brain growth is complete by 2 years of age.

Most neurological disabilities in childhood result from congenital malformation:

- The fusing process of the neural tube is critical in preventing birth defects such as spina bifida, brain injury, or infection.
- Positive reflexes in a newborn are a good indication of neurological health. A decreased level of consciousness may be an indication of a neurological problem.
- Myelinization of nerve tracts accelerate after birth following the cephalocaudal and proximodistal sequence. This allows for more complex neurological and motor function as the infant grows.

NERVOUS SYSTEM DISORDERS

CNS dysfunction may be detected by a neurologic check. Assessment of pupil reflexes, level of consciousness, balance, peripheral reflexes, and coordination can provide helpful data in determining normal from abnormal.

Reye's Syndrome

Description

- An acute noninflammatory encephalopathy and hepatopathy that follows a viral infection in children

- There is a relationship between the use of aspirin (acetylsalicylic acid) during a viral flu, chicken pox, or illness
- Some studies show that a genetic metabolic defect triggers Reye's Syndrome

Manifestations

- Liver cell destruction causes an accumulation of ammonia in the blood; assess for bleeding
- Cerebral edema causing an increase in intracranial pressure (ICP) may alter the level of consciousness, cause seizure activity, or lead to a coma

Diagnostic Criteria

- Blood tests confirming abnormal liver function
- Symptoms of diarrhea, hypoglycemia, tachypnea with apneic episodes, and seizures occurring 1 week after a respiratory illness

Interventions

- The earlier the treatment, the better the chance of recovery
- Immunization for varicella has helped to decrease the incidence of Reye's syndrome
- Reduce intracranial pressure and maintain a patent airway
- Apply oxygen; monitor fluid balance; obtain neurological checks with vital signs

=======*FAST FACTS in a NUTSHELL*

Instruct on improving the public awareness of avoiding salicylate administration to children under 19 years of age and advise to check labels for medications containing salicylate, such as Alka-Seltzer, Dristan, Ecotrin, Kaopectate, Maalox, and Pepto-Bismol.

Meningitis

Meningitis is the inflammation of the meninges, including the covering of the brain and spinal cord.

- Bacterial meningitis is a purulent or pus-forming bacteria causing a thick exudate that surrounds the meninges and adjacent structures
- Meningococcal or viral meningitis is contagious, with the main causative agent being *Haemophilus influenzae*

Description

- Organisms invade the meninges indirectly by way of the bloodstream (sepsis) from various infections throughout the body

Manifestations

- Mainly result from intracranial irritation and include severe headache, drowsiness, delirium, irritability, restlessness, fever, vomiting, and nuccal rigidity
- A classic high-pitched cry is noted in infants; seizures are common
- In severe cases, an involuntary arching of the back caused by muscle contractions is noted

Diagnostic Criteria

- Confirmed by examination of the cerebrospinal fluid (CSF) obtained through a spinal tap; cloudy fluid is abnormal
- In the CSF, a high white cell count, increase in protein, and a decrease in glucose is characteristic

Interventions

- Place child in isolation (see Appendix A, Droplet Precautions section) until 24 hours after intravenous antibiotic therapy; restore fluid and electrolyte balance
- Frequent neurologic checks, vital signs, and intake and output are required; a sedative for restlessness or an anticonvulsant may be administered. The child may be oversensitive to stimuli, thus the room should be dimly lit and quiet; speak in a soft voice
- Dexamethasone may be administered to reduce complications of bacterial meningitis

Brain Tumor

Brain tumors are the second-most common type of neoplasm in children. Most occur in the lower part of the brain (cerebellum or brainstem). Brain tumors are most common in school-age children.

Description

- A mass of tissue that is formed from an accumulation of abnormal cells
- Abnormal cells will be either benign or malignant

Manifestations

- Relate directly to the location and size of the tumor
- Increased intracranial pressure (ICP) with the hallmark symptoms of headache, vomiting, drowsiness, and seizure activity
- Nystagmus—constant jerky movements of the eyeball
- Papilledema—edema of the optic nerve
- Ataxia, head tilt, behavioral changes
- Vital sign changes occur when the tumor presses on the brainstem

Diagnostic Criteria

- Determined by clinical manifestations
- Computed tomography (CT), magnetic resonance imaging (MRI), and electroencephalogram (EEG)
- Biopsy and analysis of the abnormal tissue

Interventions

- Surgery, chemotherapy, and radiation preparation
- Preoperative care: Explain procedure; use atraumatic care techniques when providing care, such as shaving all or part of the head
- Postoperative care: Pain management; incisional assessment and care; preparation for further treatment required

Seizures

Most commonly observed neurologic dysfunction in children with sudden, intermittent periods of altered consciousness that last seconds to minutes. Physical care is similar with the varied types of seizures.

- Febrile seizures:
  - Common between 6 months and 5 years; genetic predisposition
  - Response to a rise in temperature often above 38.8° C (102° F); cause of fever needs to be ruled out
  - Administer antipyretics; use cooling measures such as having the child lightly dressed; tepid sponge bath (discontinue if shivering occurs); apply oxygen
  - Rectal or oral diazepam (Valium) for recurrent febrile seizures
  - Excellent prognosis; support child and parents in a calming tone of voice
- Status epilepticus:
  - Prolonged seizure that does not respond to treatment for 30 minutes or more; safety is the main concern
  - Can result in brain hypoxia; apply oxygen
  - Commonly caused by abruptly discontinuing medications or a generalized infection

Epilepsy

Involves a variety of neurologic and physical symptoms including:

- Period of unconsciousness; decreased awareness; or a dazed, confused state
- Recurrent sudden, periodic attacks of unconsciousness/impaired consciousness
- Contractions (tonic movements)
- Relaxation (clonic movement)
- May have alternating tonic/clonic movement of the muscles
- Staring episodes

Description

- Disorder of the central nervous system in which the neuron or nerve cells discharge in an abnormal way
- Can be focal or diffuse

- Client symptoms: Record seizure details such as aura, beginning of seizure, seizure manifestations, length of time of seizure activity, status during postictal period
- EEG to measure brain waves
- Monitor therapeutic range of prescribed anticonvulsant therapy

Seizure Type	Manifestations	Nursing Interventions
Tonic/clonic	• Shrill cry, fall risk, rigidity, aura, muscle jerking, shallow irregular breathing, loss of bowel and bladder control • Postictal period includes confusion, lethargy, sleep; return to full consciousness	• Ensure safety • Maintain a patent airway by turning on left side, loosening clothing • Speak in a calm tone, reassuring client • If seizures last more than 5 minutes, call 911
Absence (most common in children)	• Blank stare, steady distant gaze; rapid blinking or chewing motion • Begins and ends abruptly; lasts only a few seconds • Unaware of surroundings but quickly returns to being alert once seizure has passed • Learning difficulties if not recognized and treated	• Ensure safety • Speak in a calm tone, reassuring client • No emergency attention required; refer for medical evaluation
Partial	• Jerking may occur in one area of the body and progress to other areas, with the client being able to prevent movements; client may be awake and aware	• Ensure safety • Speak in a calm, reassuring tone • No emergency treatment unless seizure becomes generalized

(continued)

(continued)

Seizure Type	Manifestations	Nursing Interventions
Complex partial	• Begins with blank stare, chewing motion • Unresponsive and may be dazed and mumble; no memory of incident • Actions are clumsy, odd • Consistent actions/behavior with each seizure	• Ensure safety • Speak in a calm, reassuring tone • No emergency treatment; stay with client until aware of surroundings
Atonic seizures	• Jerking movements most frequently occurring in the morning; suddenly collapses • After a minute the client is able to stand and walk	• Ensure safety; assist client to the floor • Speak in a calm reassuring tone

Common misinformation regarding seizure care: Place something hard in mouth, hold tongue down so it cannot be swallowed, provide liquids, restrain person to ensure safety.

FAST FACTS in a NUTSHELL

A ketogenic diet is often prescribed for children who do not respond well to anticonvulsant therapy. The diet places the body in a ketoacidotic state.
The diet focuses on:

• High fat intake
• Low carbohydrates
• Adequate amount of protein

Cerebral Palsy

A group of permanent disorders inhibiting the normal development of movement and posture. There are four types, each causing activity limitations attributed to nonprogressive disturbances occurring in the developing fetal or infant brain.

- Spastic: Damage to the cortex of the brain
- Athetoid: Damage to the basal nuclei
- Ataxic:Damage to the cerebellum
- Mixed: Damage can occur in multiple areas, most commonly in the cortex and basal nuclei

Description

- Sensation and communication difficulties secondary to damage to areas of the brain, causing musculoskeletal problems
- May have normal intelligence or be mentally handicapped

Manifestations

- Manifestations (musculoskeletal/intelligence) range from mild to severe depending upon amount and location of brain damage
- In infancy, may see feeding problems, seizures, developmental delays (milestones not achieved), reflex abnormalities, spasticity of muscles, involuntary tension and twitching of muscles; characteristic appearance is legs crossed and toes pointed inward on ambulation

Diagnostic Criteria

- Genetic testing
- MRI
- Clinical manifestations

Interventions

- Assist client to perform at highest level of ability; encourage community resources
- Administer botulinum toxin for treatment of spasticity; implanted pump of baclofen
- Physical therapy to prevent contracture; maintain splints, monitor skin integrity

Intracranial Hemorrhage

An intracranial hemorrhage is the most common type of birth injury resulting most commonly from trauma during the birth process or anoxia. It occurs most often in the preterm infant due to fragile blood vessels.

Description

- An intracranial hemorrhage occurs when blood vessels within the skull are broken and bleeding into the confined skull occurs, causing an increase in pressure
- Occurs at a specific location, causing neurologic deficits

Manifestations

- Signs of neurologic compromise occur either suddenly or gradually; altered level of consciousness and oval-shaped pupils can be an early indication
- Signs of intracranial pressure include poor muscle tone, high-pitched cry, lethargy, poor sucking reflex, respiratory distress/cyanosis including Cheyne-Stokes respiratory pattern, muscle jerks, convulsions, forceful vomiting
- Opisthotonic posturing: An involuntary arching of the back and extension of the neck seen in pediatric clients with brain injury or meningeal irritation
- Fontanelles in infants appear tense and bounding

Diagnostic Criteria

- Neurologic examination
- CT scan of the head

Interventions

- Initiate interventions to decrease intracranial pressure:
  - Elevate head of bed 30 degrees
  - Anticipate administration of mannitol intravenously
  - Initiate interventions to assist the client in avoiding the Valsalva maneuver
  - Meet needs quickly to avoid crying or straining

Neural Tube Defects

Neural tube defects are commonly caused by failure of the neural tube to close at the top or lower end of the spinal cord. Emotional support of the parents and acceptance of the infant is essential.

Description

The two defects include:

- Hydrocephalus characterized by an increase of CSF within the ventricles of the brain
- Spina bifida, a group of central nervous system disorders characterized by malformation of the spinal cord

Manifestations

Defect	Manifestations
Hydrocephalus ■ Communicating: CSF is not obstructed in the ventricles but is inadequately reabsorbed in the subarachnoid space ■ Noncommunicating (obstructive): Results from the obstruction of CSF flow from the ventricles to the subarachnoid space ■ Can be congenital or acquired	• Signs depend on time of onset and the severity of the imbalance • Classic sign is an increased head size; may need a cesarean section if seen prenatally • Fontanelles bulge; skin shiny; veins dilated • "Setting sun" sign; i.e., sclera seen above the pupils • In advanced cases, body becomes thin; muscle tone poor; shrill, high-pitched cry; vomiting/anorexia; irritable with convulsions • In an older child, the predominant sign is headache

Spina bifida
■ Occulta (hidden): Minor, opening is small and there is no protrusion, often goes undetected except for a tuft of hair
■ Cystica (sac or cyst): Development of a cystic mass in the midline of the opening in the spine; two types:
  ■ Meningocele: Protrusion of membranes and CSF
  ■ Meningomyelocele: Protrusion of the membranes and spinal cord through the opening
	• Physical abnormality of the spine
	• Paralysis of the legs
	• Poor control of bowel and bladder
	• Hydrocephalus is a common complication

Diagnostic Criteria

- Transillumination: The inspection of a cavity or organ by passing a light through its walls; useful to visualize fluid. A ring of light is normal but a large halo effect is not.
- Daily head circumference.
- EEG, CT scanning, MRI of the brain to visualize ventricles.
- A ventricular tap with CSF analysis and draining.

FAST FACTS in a NUTSHELL

The American Academy of Pediatrics (2014) recommends the daily intake of folic acid 0.4 mg for women before conception as it can reduce the risk of neural tube defects.

Interventions

Defect	Nursing Interventions

Hydrocephalus	• Administer acetazolamide/furosemide per order to reduce the production of CSF
	• Offer support throughout surgical treatment and shunt placement
	  ▪ *Preoperative*: Change position frequently to prevent skin breakdown; use lamb's wool
	  ▪ Support head; assess fontanelles
	  ▪ Organize care to minimize nausea, fatigue
	  ▪ *Postoperative*: Assess for signs of increased intracranial pressure
	  ▪ Pain management/signs of infection at the suture line
	  ▪ Semi-Fowler's position to promote drainage of ventricles
	• Monitor brain function

Spina bifida • The higher the defect on the spine, the greater the neurological defect	• Preoperative: Assess sac for any leakage; cover with sterile saline dressing; use prone position • Postoperative: Assess surgical incision; prevent infection; position in side-lying position • Instruct on interventions allowing easier management of disabilities; minimize the disability

(continued)

Defect	Nursing Interventions
	• Instruct on braces, crutches, and walking devices; range-of-motion exercises
	• Encourage support groups; respite care
	• Teach bowel training and bladder management, including self-catheterization
	• Assess for latex allergy

Down's Syndrome

One of the most common chromosomal abnormalities. Parental age is a factor, with the father's age being over age 55 and the mother's age being over 35. Birth defects range from mild to severe retardation and generally some physical abnormalities.

Description

• Trisomy 21 syndrome accounts for 95% of clients; three no. 21 chromosomes rather than two occur
• Physical features

Manifestations

• Physical features, present at birth, are close-set and upward slanting eyes, small head, rounded face, flat nose, protruding tongue that interferes with sucking, and mouth breathing
• Simian crease (straight line across palm)
• Physical growth may be slow; muscles may be hypotonic including lungs; positioning or holding the infant may be difficult; respiratory infection with mucus accumulation common
• Congenital heart deformities are common
• Intelligence quotients (IQs) may range from very low to below average

Diagnostic Criteria

• Screening can be completed during the first trimester of pregnancy via an ultrasound
• A serum alfa fetal protein (AFP) test, unconjugated estriol (UE), a placenta hormone (inhibin-A), and human chorionic

gonadotropin (hCG) can be administered during the second trimester of pregnancy
- Positive test results from the first or second trimester can indicate the need for an amniocentesis
- A chromosome analysis will confirm the specific type

Interventions

- Physical assessment focusing on the cardiac and respiratory system
- Encourage the child to answer questions and complete personal care independently as able, living to his or her full potential
- Support parents; take time to comment on positive characteristics of the child; refer to a support group

REFERENCES AND FURTHER READING

Hockenberry, M., & Wilson, D. (2013). *Wong's essentials of pediatric nursing* (9th ed.). St. Louis, MO: Elsevier.

Leifer, G. (2011). *Introduction to maternity & pediatric nursing* (6th ed.). St. Louis, MO: Elsevier.

12

Skin Disorders

There are distinct integumentary system differences between the child and the adult. At birth, the alkalinity of the newborn skin increases susceptibility to infection. Newborns have less subcutaneous fat, leaving them more sensitive to heat and cold. In infants, the epidermis is thinner, blisters more easily, and is more prone to infections. The sebaceous glands in children do not become active until school age, often resulting in dry, chapped skin. Skin infections in children are more likely to result in systemic symptoms than in adults. Skin lesions and disfigurations have both a physiological and psychological component that can impact normal growth and development in the child. The pediatric nurse who understands the skin characteristics that exist in children has an increased ability to identify and assist in treating problems when they occur.

This chapter reviews:

1. Common congenital skin lesions (birthmarks)
2. Acquired skin lesions in children
3. Skin alterations associated with burns
4. Fungal infections in children

CONGENITAL LESIONS/BIRTH MARKS

Discolorations of the skin are common findings in newborn infants. Most involve no therapy other than reassurance to parents of the benign nature. More extensive lesions require further scrutiny and may need excision when feasible.

Stork's Beak Marks/Stork Bites

Description

- Reddish or pink patches that are often found above the hairline at the nape of the neck, eyelids, or between the eyes

Manifestations/Diagnosis

- Caused by collections of capillary blood vessels close to the skin

Interventions

- No intervention necessary; usually fade with time

Mongolian Spots

Description

- Bluish discolorations on the skin. Resemble bruises. Usually on sacral and gluteal areas but can be found on other areas

Manifestations/Diagnosis

- More common in African Americans, Native Americans, and Asians

Interventions

- No intervention necessary; fade during pre-school years

Port-Wine Stain

Description

- Port-wine stain is a permanent, flat, dark pink or reddish-purple mark

Manifestations/Diagnosis

- Varies in size and location. Does not blanch with pressure.
- Thickens, darkens, and proportionally enlarges as the child grows
- May be associated with structural malformations such as glaucoma or leptomeningeal angiomatosis (tumors of blood or lymph vessels in the pia-arachnoid) and bony or muscular overgrowth

Interventions

- Children with port-wine stains on the eyelids, forehead, or cheeks should be monitored with periodic ophthalmologic exams, neurologic imaging, and measurement of extremities
- It can be removed via flashlamp-pumped pulse-dye laser

Strawberry Mark/Strawberry Hemangioma

Description

- Collection of capillaries at the skin surface
- More common in females

Manifestations/Diagnosis

- Raised, bright red, rubbery nodules with a rough surface and well-defined margins
- May appear within several weeks after birth
- Enlarges during the first year of life then stops growing

Interventions

- None needed. Involutes spontaneously (between ages 5 and 12 years)

Café-au-Lait Spot

Description

- Permanent, pale brown areas of increased melanin in the skin anywhere on the body

Manifestations/Diagnosis

- Usually 0.8 to 8 inches in size with irregular borders
- May fade with age
- May be a marker for systemic neurofibromatosis (tumors of the nervous system)

Interventions

- Darker, more extensive lesions need to be scrutinized
- Excision of lesion when feasible

Congenital Nevus

Description

- A large, dark-colored mole that typically appears on the scalp or trunk of the body

Manifestations/Diagnosis

- Can range in size from less than 1 cm to 20 cm across, covering large areas
- Children with a congenital nevus, especially those with a large-sized nevus, are at an increased risk of developing skin cancer as adults

Interventions

- Dark brown or black macules can become more numerous with age
- Risk for developing malignant melanoma

OTHER SKIN LESIONS

Acne Vulgaris

Description

- An inflammation of the sebaceous glands and hair follicles in the skin

- The most common skin problem treated during adolescence, with peak incidence during middle to late adolescence
- Hormonal influence (testosterone) during puberty stimulates the sebaceous glands of the skin to enlarge, or produce oil, and plug the pores

Manifestations

- Usually seen on the chin, cheeks, and forehead
- Can develop on the chest and upper back and shoulders
- Consists of open comedones (blackheads) and closed comedones (whiteheads)
- Whiteheads cause the inflammatory process of acne resulting in formation of pustules, papules, nodules, and cysts

Interventions

- No known link to dietary intake
- Goal of treatment is to prevent scarring and promote self-image
- Gentle skin cleansing; avoid cosmetics containing lanolin, petrolatum, oils, and alcohol-based products
- Sunshine
- Benzoyl peroxide, an antibacterial agent, is an effective first-line agent
- Tretinoin (Retin-A) manages comedonal acne
- Topical/oral antibiotics
- Isotretinoin (Accutane) for severe putulocystic acne
- Dermabrasion can be used to minimize scarring
- Can lead to physical and emotional scarring

FAST FACTS in a NUTSHELL

Accutane has teratogenic effects and is contraindicated in young women, without the use of effective contraceptives. Behavior and mood changes, including suicidal ideation, are added side effects of this drug.

Burns

Description

- Leading cause of accidental deaths in the home for children ages 1 to 4 years of age
- Tissue injury caused by thermal heat, chemicals, electricity, or radiation
- The child's skin is thinner than adult skin, leading to more serious depth of burn at lower temperatures and shorter exposure time
- Children have a larger body surface area, which results in greater fluid, electrolyte, and heat loss
- Increased basal metabolic rate results in greater protein and calorie needs
- Immature immune system predisposes the child to greater infection complications
- Greater risk for scarring due to more elasticity of the skin in children

Manifestations/Diagnosis

- Classification of burn begins with total body surface area (TBSA)
  - **Lund Browder Method** is a more accurate method for children as compared to **Rule of Nine or Palm Method** (Manchester Royal Infirmary, 2009).
  - Methods for assessing figures can be accessed at: www.ncbi.nlm.nih.gov/pmc/articles/PMC449823/
  - If body surface area is greater than 10%, intravenous fluid resuscitation is necessary
- Depth of burn
  - Partial thickness
    - First-degree burn: Only epidermis has been damaged
      - Erythematous, blanches, painful to touch, hypersensitive, uncomfortable
    - Second-degree burn: Epidermis and superficial (papillary) dermis are damaged
      - Erythematous, wet, and often blistering; extreme pain
  - Full thickness
    - Third-degree burn: Epidermis, papillary and deep dermis, and different depths of subcutaneous tissue are damaged
      - Painless
      - Hard, leathery eschar; may appear charred

– Fourth-degree burn: Extensive damage to deep structures (muscle or bone)
  – Will not heal, requires amputation
- Chemical burns: Cannot assess until chemicals removed
- Electrical burns: Have entrance and exit wounds and cause greater internal damage

FAST FACTS in a NUTSHELL

Silvadene is great for surface wounds but does not penetrate well. Always debride the area and cleanse to remove old layers of the medication before application. Do NOT apply silver products to the face; can cause skin color changes.

Interventions

- Remove source of heat, stop the burning
- Assess for inhalation injury first and secure airway!
- Assess zones of injury and prevent further vasoconstriction
- Prevent hypovolemic shock and establish IV site
- Fluid resuscitation in 20% TBSA burns or greater
- Escharotomies and fasciotomies to prevent further compromised circulation/breathing
- Hydrotherapy for debridement
- Application of topicals to minimize drying, facilitate healing, and minimize risk of infection
- Skin grafting (allograft, xenograft, or synthetic skin covering)
- Keep wounds clean and dry
- Temperature control
- Pain management
- Standard precautions
- Transfer to burn center

Atopic Dermatitis/Infantile Eczema

Description

- Inflammation of genetically hypersensitive skin
- Rarely seen in breastfed infants until foods added to diet
- Familial history of allergies; eczema, asthma, food allergies, or allergic rhinitis

- Usually begins at 2 to 6 months of age with spontaneous remission by 3 years of age
- Emotional factors; methods of coping may be a factor

Manifestations

- Local vasodilation progresses to *spongiosis* (breakdown of dermal cells and formation of intradermal vesicles)
- Distribution on cheeks, scalp, trunk, and extensor surfaces
- Appearance of lesions: Erythema, vesicles, papules, weeping, oozing, crusting, and scaling
- Chronic scratching produces *lichenification* (coursening of skin folds)

FAST FACTS in a NUTSHELL

Question: When is the best time to apply emollient preparations to the skin?

Answer: It is imperative that the emollient preparation be applied immediately after bathing (while the skin is still slightly moist) to prevent drying.

Diagnosis

- Based on history and morphologic findings

Interventions

- Hydrate the skin via emollient application
- Relieve pruritus with tepid colloid bath (cornstarch or baking soda) and antihistamines
- Reduce flares of inflammation with topical steroids
- Prevent secondary infection by keeping nails trimmed
- Some children will develop asthma or allergic rhinitis/hay fever

Impetigo Contagiosa

Description

- An infectious disease of the skin caused by staphylococci or group-A beta-hemolytic streptococci.
- Newborns are susceptible due to low resistance to skin bacteria.

Manifestations

- Bullous form: Lesions of red papules that become vesicles or pustules surrounded by reddened area
- When blisters break, the surface is raw and weeping
- Lesions may occur anywhere but mostly found around the nose, mouth, and most areas of the body
- Contagious and spreads easily

====================================*FAST FACTS in a NUTSHELL*

Impetigo is a bacterial infection that is often caused by MRSA or group-A beta-hemolytic streptococci. To prevent complications of beta-hemolytic streptococcal infections (such as nephritis), impetigo should be treated with antibiotics.

Diagnosis

- Based on findings

Interventions

- Prevention: Prompt attention to minor cuts and bites
- Systemic antibiotics and wash lesions several times per day
- Prevent spread of infection with frequent handwashing and good hygiene practices

Scabies

Description

- Contagious parasitic infestation with the "itch mite"
- Spread by close personal contact
- Adult female mite burrows under the skin and lays eggs

Manifestations

- Burrows are sometimes seen under the skin and between fingers
- Itching is intense and increased at night
- Vesicles and pustules can occur in children
- Thrives in moist body folds but in young children can appear on head, palms, and soles of feet

FAST FACTS in a NUTSHELL

Question: What amount of medication should be prescribed in the treatment of scabies?

Answer: Because of the length of time between infestation and physical symptoms ranges from 30 to 60 days, all persons who were in close contact with the affected child need treatment. Allow 2 oz for each adult and 1oz for each child.

Diagnosis

- Based on findings and reports of infestations

Interventions

- Application of scabicide; the drug of choice in children and infants older than 2 months is permethrin 5% cream (Elimite)
- Treat all persons in close direct contact with the child

DERMATOPHYTOSES OR FUNGAL INFECTIONS OF THE SKIN

Fungal infections are caused by several closely related fungi that have a preference for invading the stratum corneum, the hair, and the nails. Transmission can be via person to person or animal to person.

Tinea Capitis/Ringworm of the Scalp

Description

- Fungal infection of the scalp
- Mostly seen in school-age children

Manifestations

- Circular patches of alopecia (hair loss)
- Hair loses pigment and may break off
- Papules and pustules can progress to red scales

Teaching points specific to oral griseofulvin medication use should include the following:

- Take with high-fat food to reduce GI irritation and increase absorption.
- There is a need for periodic testing for leukopenia, liver, and renal function with long-term use.

Diagnosis

- Based on history and appearance

Interventions

- Treated with oral medication: griseofulvin (Fulvicin, Grisactin)
- Selenium shampoos
- Avoid exposure to the sun
- Treatment may take 8 to 12 weeks

Tinea Pedis/Athlete's Foot

Description

- Ringworm infection of the feet

Manifestations

- Lesions are located between the toes, on the instep, and on the soles
- Accompanied with pruritus
- More common in preadolescents and adolescents

Diagnosis

- Based on history and appearance and microscopic scrapings

Interventions

- Topical application of antifungal preparations
- Oral griseofulvin may be given
- Condition is aggravated by heat and moisture; dry between toes and wear clean socks

Tinea Corporis/Ringworm of the Skin

Description

- Fungal infection of the skin

Manifestations

- Oval, scaly, inflamed ring with a clear center
- Seen on face, neck, arms, and hands

FAST FACTS in a NUTSHELL

Ringworm is spread through direct contact with household pets, especially cats. All household pets should be examined for the disorder.

Diagnosis

- Based on history and appearance

Interventions

- Local application of antifungal preparation such as haloprogin, tolnaftate, miconazole, or clotrimazole for 1 to 2 weeks or until no lesions are seen
- Griseofulvin for more severe cases

Tinea Cruris/Jock Itch

Description

- Fungal infection of the groin area

Description

• Fungal infection of the nails

CONCLUSION

Presentation and location of lesions on the skin may produce stress and anxiety in the child and parent. Prevention of permanent scarring is the desired outcome and can present a challenge to the pediatric nurse.

REFERENCES AND FURTHER READING

Hockenberry, M., & Wilson, D. (2013). *Wong's essentials of pediatric nursing* (9th ed.). St. Louis, MO: Elsevier.

Leifer, G. (2011). *Introduction to maternity & pediatric nursing* (6th ed.). St. Louis, MO: Elsevier.

Manchester Royal Infirmary. (2009, August). *Assessing the size of burns in patients: Which method works best.* Retrieved from http://bestbets.org/bets/bet.php?id=957

U.S. Department of Health and Human Services. (2013, August). *Burn triage and treatment: Thermal injuries.* Retrieved from http://www.remm.nlm.gov/burns.htm

13

Respiratory Disorders

Respiratory disorders are the most common causes of illness and hospitalization in children. Respiratory disorders range from mild and self-limiting to life-threatening. The human respiratory system provides oxygen to each cell of the body but also removes body wastes, filters out infectious agents, and provides air needed for speech. Respiratory dysfunction tends to be more severe in children than adults and is a frequent cause of emergency department visits. Pediatric respiratory health is promoted through prevention, early detection, treatment of disorders, and education efforts.

This chapter reviews:

1. Common pediatric respiratory disorders
2. Etiology of pediatric respiratory disorders
3. Specific care of pediatric clients with respiratory disorders

VARIATIONS IN PEDIATRIC ANATOMY AND PHYSIOLOGY

Newborns are obligatory nose breathers until 1 month of age. They breathe through their mouth only when crying. Newborns have less mucous production, making them more susceptible to infection. Throughout childhood, infants/preschoolers have larger tongues, tonsils, and adenoids, which can cause airway obstruction even in the absence of disease. Also, the lumen of the airway is smaller, which makes the presence of even a small amount of edema or mucus a concern for respiratory compromise. A short, narrow airway can allow infection to travel quickly to the lower airways.

UPPER RESPIRATORY TRACT DISORDERS

The common cold is the most common upper respiratory infection (URI) or nasopharyngitis. URIs are more common in the winter. It is not unusual for children to have 6 to 9 colds per year. Spontaneous resolution occurs in 7 to 10 days.

An upper respiratory tract disorder is a disorder of the:

- Nose/nasal cavity/sinuses
- Pharynx/larynx
- Upper trachea

ETIOLOGY

The causes of a URI include rhinoviruses, parainfluenza, and the respiratory syncytial virus (RSV). Most URIs are thought to be a result of a virus but complications can include secondary bacterial infections of the ears, nose, throat, sinuses, and/or lungs. Infectious agents have easy access to the middle ear through the short and open eustachian tubes of infants and young children.

It is important to note that viral illnesses are treated symptomatically and bacterial infections are treated with antibiotics. Research stresses the selective use of antibiotics throughout a lifetime.

Some risk factors are known to increase incidence of URIs:

- School or daycare attendance
- Lack of good handwashing
- Second-hand smoke
- Contact with other persons who have a URI
- Allergies

Common Cold

Description

- A relatively harmless disorder that usually is self-limiting
- May lead to a secondary infection, most commonly an ear infection

Manifestations

- Nasal inflammation, rhinorrhea, cough, sneezing, and nasal quality of voice
- Little or no fever associated
- Mild fatigue, slight achiness

===*FAST FACTS in a NUTSHELL*

Many parents seek medical care for symptoms of the common cold in children. The common cold is treated symptomatically with age-appropriate dosages of analgesics and symptom relievers. If no secondary infection is present, typically no antibiotic is prescribed.

Diagnostic Criteria

- Physical exam and assessment of presenting symptoms
- Diagnostic testing such as inner ear evaluation, throat culture, or chest x-ray to rule out secondary infections

Interventions

- Increase fluid intake, keeping throat moist and preventing dehydration; use a cool moist humidifier
- Saline nose drops; blue bulb syringe to remove mucus
- Medications include analgesics and symptomatic treatments for congestion, cough, and runny nose
- Excellent prognosis

Influenza

Description

- A highly contagious viral infection typically contracted in the winter
- Influenza types A and B are most common
- Most commonly transmitted by air or on objects; most contagious period is 24 hours prior to noticeable symptoms

Manifestations

- Fever, muscle aches, sore throat, headache, nonproductive cough
- Symptoms usually last a few days; however, severe illness and death can occur

FAST FACTS in a NUTSHELL

Question: In which instance would children be unable to obtain the FluMist nasal spray vaccine?

Answer: The FluMist nasal spray vaccine is administered to healthy children and adolescents (ages 2 to 17 years). As with other live vaccines, children who are immunosuppressed or taking immunosuppressant medications are excluded.

Diagnostic Criteria

- Physical exam and assessment of presenting symptoms
- If necessary, a flu culture (rapid flu test) confirms diagnosis

Interventions

- Two antiviral medications are used to prevent influenza in children; both are taken at the onset of symptoms
- Treatment is symptomatic depending upon conditions exhibited
- Increase fluid intake; bedrest
- The drug of choice is acetaminophen

Description

- Inflammation and pain of the throat mucosa/tonsils or adenoids. May also include symptoms of enlarged lymph nodes, fever, cough, congestion. White patches may be noted on tonsils and adenoids with inflammation that limits breathing
- May be viral or bacterial
- Group A *Streptococcus* (*Strep* throat) is common and may lead to peritonsillar or retropharyngeal abscesses
- Onset of symptoms is abrupt
- Viral pharyngitis may resolve in a few days; *Strep* throat requires completion of antibiotic therapy

Manifestations

- Sore throat with redness of the pharynx, possible tonsillar exudate, and white strawberry tongue coating
- Fever, headache, cervical lymphadenopathy, and hoarse quality to voice
- Adenoids can be inflamed and hypertrophied but difficult to see due to location
- Difficulty breathing or swallowing can occur; snoring may occur

══ FAST FACTS in a NUTSHELL

Recipe for a saline gargle:

8 oz water and ½ teaspoon of table salt

Diagnostic Criteria

- Physical exam and assessment of presenting symptoms
- Rapid test or throat culture; throat culture may be positive for *Streptococcus*
- Complete blood count with differential

Interventions

- Penicillin is typically prescribed for *Strep* throat
- Saline gargles are soothing; acetaminophen or ibuprofen for pain

- Encourage popsicles, cool liquids, and ice chips to maintain hydration
- Removal of the tonsils or adenoids may be indicated with recurrent infections or hypertrophy; be alert to frequent swallowing indicating hemorrhage postoperatively
- Discard old toothbrush to prevent reinfection
- Children must be on antibiotics for 24 hours before they are considered noncontagious
- Prognosis is excellent

Epiglottitis

Description

- Inflammation of the epiglottis most often caused by *Haemophilus influenzae* type b.
- Occurs in children between the ages of 1 and 7 and may be life-threatening
- Rapid onset

Manifestations

- High fever
- Characterized by dysphagia, drooling, anxiety, and irritability
- Respiratory distress and death may occur if airway becomes obstructed
- The child may refuse to lie down or speak

FAST FACTS in a NUTSHELL

Nurses perform detailed physical assessments; however, when caring for a client with epiglottitis, it is essential that the nurse forego visualization of the client's throat. Placing anything in the mouth to assess the throat could cause the inflamed area to spasm and obstruct, causing respiratory distress.

Diagnostic Criteria

- Physical examination analyzing symptoms presented
- Lateral neck radiography to note swelling

Interventions

- Airway maintenance and support; never leave the child unattended
- Place on 100% supplemental oxygen; IV antibiotic therapy
- If complete airway obstruction occurs, a tracheostomy may be required
- Administration of the *Haemophilus influenzae* type b (Hib) vaccine
- Keep the child calm
- Do not place in a supine position; allow the child to determine a position of comfort

Croup/Laryngotracheobronchitis

Description

- Inflammation and edema of the larynx, trachea, and bronchi, which occurs as a result of a virus
- Mucous production and narrowing of airways can cause stridor
- Self-limiting, lasts only 3 to 5 days
- Most commonly affects children 3 months to 3 years

Manifestations

- Voice hoarseness and a barking cough
- Inflammation of the airway with suprasternal retractions
- Onset is sudden and usually at night
- Complications are rare

Diagnostic Criteria

- Physical examination analyzing symptoms presented
- A lateral neck radiography to rule out epiglottitis

Interventions

- Corticosteroids are used to decrease inflammation
- Racemic epinephrine aerosols to decrease edema
- Encourage rest, semi-Fowler's position, and increase fluid intake
- Use humidified air via a cool mist humidifier or steamy shower

LOWER RESPIRATORY TRACT DISORDERS

Pediatric disorders that affect the lower respiratory tract can be short- or long-term conditions depending upon the cause. Short-term conditions cause acute inflammation of the bronchial tubes or lungs including pneumonia, bronchitis, and bronchiolitis. Long-term conditions occur when underlying disorders cause swelling and inflammation for an extended period of time. Asthma and cystic fibrosis are examples.

A lower respiratory tract disorder is a disorder of the:

- Lower trachea
- Bronchi
- Bronchioles
- Alveoli

ETIOLOGY

Viral infections are the most common cause of short-term lower respiratory tract infections, many times spreading from infections of the upper respiratory tract . Long-term lower respiratory tract infections are related to genetic diseases or allergen triggers.

DIAGNOSES

Asthma

Description

- Caused by an inflammation and narrowing of the airways
- The muscles surrounding the airways tighten and the lining swells
- Airway hyperresponsiveness can occur due to allergens, air pollution, family history, or viral infection
- The most common chronic illness of childhood; a long-term complication of airway remodeling occurs from frequent exacerbations
- Acute complications include status asthmaticus and respiratory compromise

Manifestations

- Symptoms vary from mild, only occurring with exercise, to severe, interfering with activities of daily living
- Cough with or without sputum, especially at night
- Shortness of breath with wheezing and intercostal retractions
- Chest tightness with recurrent periods of wheezing

=== *FAST FACTS in a NUTSHELL*

A child who is in respiratory distress is frightened and often clings to the parent for safety and reassurance. Allow the parent to provide as much support and care as possible without interfering with nursing actions. Direct all instructions to the parent.

Diagnostic Criteria

- Physical examination analyzing symptoms presented
- Recurrent symptoms of shortness of breath, wheezing, and cough
- Pulse oximetry, blood gases, pulmonary functions test, and chest x-ray
- Tracking of peak flow meter data provides diagnostic and treatment information
- Allergy testing

Interventions

- Early and aggressive asthma treatment is essential to interrupt symptom progression
- Medication therapy including anti-inflammatory medications, bronchodilators, and steroids administered orally, intravenously, or by inhalation
- Identify symptom triggers and eliminate; do not smoke
- Provide stepwise approach to asthma management
- Teach the usefulness of asthma management by using a peak flow meter

Bronchiolitis/Respiratory Syncytial Virus

Description

- Bronchiolitis is an acute inflammatory process of the bronchioles and small bronchi. Bronchiolitis is nearly always caused by a viral pathogen or respiratory syncytial virus, which accounts for the majority of cases of bronchiolitis
- The peak incidence is in the winter and spring
- The frequency and severity of RSV infection decrease with age (especially for those 6 months and younger) and are localized to the upper respiratory tract after toddlerhood. Prematurity and multiple births are predisposing factors.
- Contagious in nature

Manifestations

- Rhinorrhea, pharyngitis, intermittent fever, cough with mucous production, and wheezing. Infants may be listless and uninterested in feeding
- Deteriorating respiratory status, including an increased respiratory rate, bronchial constriction, nasal flaring, retractions, and cyanosis
- Serious alteration in gas exchange occurs with hypoxemia and carbon dioxide retention. The infant with tachypnea, significant retractions, poor oral intake, or lethargy can deteriorate quickly, to the point of requiring ventilator support

FAST FACTS in a NUTSHELL

Procedure for obtaining nasal–pharyngeal washings:
Nasal–pharyngeal washings are obtained by instilling 1 to 3 mL of normal saline via syringe in the nares and then aspirating the loosened nasal secretions for analysis.

Diagnostic Criteria

- Physical exam, including auscultation of lung fields
- Collection of nasal secretions to detect RSV

Interventions

- Note any cyanosis; apply supplemental oxygen as directed
- Nasal or nasopharyngeal suctioning as needed

- Maintain hydration via increased fluids or intravenous hydration
- Aerosolized ribavirin is recommended only in the most severely ill children
- Place in a semi-Fowler's position

Cystic Fibrosis

Description

- An autosomal recessive disorder (both parents must be carriers) that affects the lungs, pancreas, small intestine, and liver
- Abnormally thick mucus production leads to mechanical obstruction of the organs, leading to organ dysfunction
- Sweat and salivary glands excrete excessive sodium and chloride

_____ *FAST FACTS in a NUTSHELL*

A salty taste to skin when kissed is a physical characteristic that a parent can identify as a manifestation of cystic fibrosis.

Manifestations

- Abdominal pain with difficulty passing stools
- Bulky, greasy stools
- Poor weight gain
- Meconium ileus or delayed meconium in the newborn period
- Respiratory distress with adventitious breath sounds, nasal polyps, cough with sputum, and decreased oxygen saturation
- Barrel chest, nail clubbing

Diagnostic Criteria

- History of chronic respiratory infections, poor weight gain, and failure to thrive
- Sweat sodium test with results greater than 60 mEq/L; DNA testing confirms diagnosis
- Stool analysis notes presence of pancreatic enzymes
- Chest x-ray, pulmonary function test

Interventions

- Teach breathing exercises, administration of breathing treatments, chest physiotherapy, and productive coughing techniques
- Perform chest physiotherapy 1 hour before meals and 2 hours after meals, if possible; instruct on a mucus clearing device if applicable
- Promote high-calorie and high-protein nutrition with pancreatic enzymes at all meals and snacks; emphasize good oral hygiene
- Administer fat-soluble vitamins (A, D, E, K) with snacks and meals; administer Pulmozyme via nebulizer to decrease viscosity of mucus
- Monitor all blood tests including blood glucose levels
- Monitor hydration status and encourage salt intake, especially in the summer months

Pneumonia

Description

- Inflammation of the lung parenchyma; viral or bacterial
- Viral pneumonia is better tolerated by children, frequently affects the alveolar wall, and is passed from the upper respiratory tract
- In bacterial pneumonia, mucus stasis causes air trapping in the lungs. Inflammation of the alveoli results in atelectasis impairing gas exchange

FAST FACTS in a NUTSHELL

Observing the child's respiratory effort during a physical exam is an important first step in diagnosing pneumonia. The World Health Organization (WHO) respiratory rate thresholds for identifying children with pneumonia are as follows:

- Children younger than 2 months: Greater than or equal to 60 breaths/min
- Children aged 2 to 11 months: Greater than or equal to 50 breaths/min
- Children aged 12 to 59 months: Greater than or equal to 40 breaths/min

Manifestations

- Cyanosis, nasal flaring, tachypnea
- Adventitious breath sounds such as wheezes, rales, and diminished or absent breath sounds
- Low oxygen saturation levels
- Cough with or without sputum, chills, fever, shortness of breath on exertion, and chest pain
- Nausea and vomiting may occur

Diagnostic Criteria

- Physical examination analyzing symptoms presented
- Chest x-ray, complete blood count, and sputum culture
- Adventitious, especially crackles or absent breath sounds

Interventions

- Antipyretics for an elevated fever
- Antibiotics
- Elevate head of bed to promote lung aeration
- Increase fluids, administer intravenously if needed
- Obtain sputum culture before beginning antibiotic therapy, if needed

REFERENCES AND FURTHER READING

Centers for Disease Control and Prevention. (2014). *Seasonal influenza*. Retrieved from http://www.cdc.gov/flu

Hockenberry, M., & Wilson, D. (2013). *Wong's essentials of pediatric nursing* (9th ed.). St. Louis, MO: Elsevier.

Leifer, G. (2011). *Introduction to maternity & pediatric nursing* (6th ed.). St. Louis, MO: Elsevier.

14

Cardiovascular Disorders

> Cardiovascular diseases in children can be either congenital or acquired. Identification of heart defects in newborns and infants requires reliance on objective data collection, since this age group is unable to verbalize symptoms.
>
> Recognition of a heart defect in a child can be one of the most frightening experiences for any parent. The nurse needs to provide nursing management of the cardiac disorder while providing emotional support and encouragement to the parents. The nursing goals significant to the care of a child with heart disorder are to reduce the work of the heart, improve respirations, maintain proper nutrition, prevent infection, reduce anxiety of the parent, and support growth and development.

This chapter reviews:

1. Common congenital heart disorders
2. Common childhood-acquired heart disorders
3. Diagnostic criteria used to identify cardiac disorders in children

CONGENITAL HEART DISEASE (CHD)

Incidence in children is approximately. 8:1,000 live births. About 50% will be symptomatic during the first year of life. The exact cause is unknown. Most are thought to be a result of multifactor inheritance (genetic and environmental).

Some risk factors that are known to increase incidence of CHD:

- Chronic illness of mother
- Alcohol consumption
- Exposure to environmental toxins/infections
- Family history of first-degree relative having defect

CHD resulting in heart anomalies are often associated with chromosomal abnormalities or congenital defects in other body systems. Down syndrome (trisomy 21) and trisomy 13 and 18 are highly correlated with congenital heart defects.

Classification of CHD is by hemodynamic classification.

- Shunting:
  - Blood flow through an abnormal opening in the heart or great vessel
  - Oxygen saturation is increased or decreased in the normally desaturated or fully saturated blood
  Blood flow:
- Normally the blood flow to the lungs through the pulmonary artery is the same as to the systemic circulation through the aorta (1:1 ratio). However, the pulmonary-to-systemic blood flow ratios can vary from normal, decreased, or increased in children with CHD

Atrial Septal Defect

Description

- Abnormal opening between atria
- More common in females
- Oxygenated blood shunts left to right (no cyanosis)

Manifestations

- Most infants and children are asymptomatic but in time may develop fatigue and dyspnea
- Palpitations, atrial dysrhythmias
- Recurrent respiratory infections (due to increased pulmonary blood flow)
- Systolic murmur; diastolic murmur with large shunts
- Rare: Heart failure (HF), stroke, or major organ damage from embolism

Diagnostic Criteria

- Physical exam and assessment of presenting symptoms
- Echocardiography, cardiac catheterization, and cardiac magnetic resonance imaging (MRI)

Interventions

- Since atrial septal defects do not close spontaneously, patching via open-heart surgery or cardiac catheterization will be necessary
- Excellent prognosis

Coarctation of the Aorta

Description

- Narrowing of the aorta near the insertion of the ductus arteriosus, which increases pressure proximal to the defect
- Pressure increased to the head, upper extremities, and the left ventricle
- Blood supply and pressure is decreased to the abdominal organs and lower extremities
- Children with this disorder are at risk for bicuspid valve stenosis later in life

Manifestations

- Symptoms are directly related to the severity of constriction
- May be asymptomatic until late childhood
- Systolic hypertension and bounding pulses in arms
- Permanent residual hypertension is related to age and time of repair
- Weak or absent femoral pulses and cool lower extremities

═══════════════════════════*FAST FACTS in a NUTSHELL*

Question: What is the characteristic sign of coarctation of the aorta?

Answer: A significant difference in blood pressure between upper extremities and lower extremities.

Diagnostic Criteria

- Physical exam and assessment of presenting symptoms
- Echocardiography, cardiac catheterization, and cardiac MRI

Interventions

- Percutaneous balloon angioplasty with stents (choice treatment for older child)
- Closed-heart surgery: Resection and anastomosis/grafting of the aorta may be necessary and is the treatment of choice in infants less than 6 months
- Monitor for signs of recurrence
- Prognosis is good

Patent Ductus Arteriosus (PDA)

Description

- Opening between aorta and pulmonary artery fails to close after birth
- Oxygenated blood from aorta flows back to pulmonary artery, increasing workload on the heart
- Common especially in premature infants and two times more common in girls

Manifestations

- Many children are clinically asymptomatic
- Continuous murmur with suprasternal thrill
- Increased pulse pressure with bounding
- Heart enlarges
- Tachypnea, poor feeding, weight gain, frequent respiratory infections, fatigue, and diaphoresis
- Premature infants: Present with heart failure (HF) and increased respiratory distress
- The degree of HF symptoms depends on the amount of left-to-right shunting

The primary focus of nursing care in an infant with patent ductus arteriosus is to prevent heart failure and pulmonary congestion. Stay alert and report any of the following early signs of heart failure: tachycardia at rest, fatigue during feeding, sweating of scalp and forehead, dyspnea, and sudden weight gain.

Diagnostic Criteria

- Physical exam and assessment of presenting symptoms
- Echocardiography, cardiac catheterization, and cardiac MRI

Interventions

- Administration of indomethacin has proven successful in closing a PDA in preterm infants and some newborns
- Video-assisted thoracoscopic surgery to ligate or clip the ductus
- Nonsurgical options include insertion of coil to occlude PDA via cardiac catheterization
- Prognosis is excellent

Tetralogy of Fallot

Description

- Tetralogy of Fallot is a congenital heart defect in which a decrease in pulmonary blood flow results in unoxygenated blood going into general circulation
- Four separate defects:
  - Stenosis of pulmonary artery (decreases blood flow to lungs)
  - Hypertrophy of right ventricle
  - Aorta displaced to right (blood from both ventricles entering)
  - Ventricular septal defect

Manifestations: Cyanotic Defect

- Pulmonary stenosis (severity) leads to greater desaturation of blood
- Tires easily, especially with exertion
- Difficulty with feeding and gaining weight
- Hypercyanotic events, chronic hypoxia with clubbing
- Harsh systolic murmur with thrill

FAST FACTS in a NUTSHELL

Cyanosis may be present at birth as reflected in a blue coloration. Therefore, the term "blue baby" is often associated with this disorder.

Diagnostic Criteria

- Physical exam and assessment of presenting symptoms
- X-ray reveals "boot shaped" heart due to poor development of pulmonary artery
- Elevated hematocrit and hemoglobin – compensates for lack of circulating O_2
- Echocardiography, cardiac catheterization, and cardiac MRI

Interventions

- Treatment is aimed to increase pulmonary blood flow to relieve hypoxia
- Blalock–Taussig procedure for newborns (temporary shunt to increase pulmonary blood flow)
- Open-heart surgery on older child with excellent results

Ventricular Septal Defect

Description

- Abnormal opening between the right and left ventricles
- Most common CHD
- Blood shunts from left to right (no cyanosis)

Manifestations

- Symptoms become apparent in first few weeks of life with larger defects and include:
  - Murmur, loud and harsh over systole
- May develop congestive heart failure with accompanied poor feeding, failure to thrive

Diagnostic Criteria

- Physical exam and assessment of presenting symptoms
- Echocardiography, cardiac catheterization, and cardiac MRI

═══════════════════════════════*FAST FACTS in a NUTSHELL*

Small ventricular septal defects often close spontaneously during the first year of life.

Interventions

- Cardiac catheterization procedure can be used for small defects
- Open-heart surgery for suture ligation or patch of larger holes
- Prognosis is excellent

ACQUIRED HEART DISEASE

Acquired heart disease is a cardiac problem that occurs *after* birth. It may be a complication of a congenital heart disease or a response to respiratory infection, sepsis, hypertension, or severe anemia.

Hyperlipidemia (Hypercholesterolemia)

Description

- Excessive lipids or cholesterol in the blood
- High cholesterol can be a familial, genetic, or lifestyle component or can be caused by secondary problems (such as hypothyroidism)

Manifestations

- A presymptomatic phase of atherosclerosis can begin in childhood

FAST FACTS in a NUTSHELL

Question: What are the acceptable, borderline, and high total cholesterol and LDL cholesterol levels in children and adolescents 2 to 19 years old?

Answer: Total cholesterol (mg/dL): Acceptable—less than 170; Borderline—170 to 199; High—200 or greater. LDL cholesterol (mg/dL): Acceptable—less than 110; Borderline—110 to 129; High—130 or greater.

Diagnostic Criteria

- Identify high-risk children:
  - Parent/grandparent with cerebrovascular and/or cardio-vascular disease
  - Parent with total cholesterol greater than 240
  - Tobacco use, decreased exercise, obesity, or high fat intake
- Analysis of blood for a full lipid profile, drawn after a 12-hour fast

Interventions

- Lifestyle modification—avoid tobacco use, increase activity level
- Nutritional counseling—heart-healthy diet for all children
- Cholesterol-lowering drugs *not* usually used in younger children

Kawasaki Disease/Syndrome (Mucocutaneous Lymph Node Syndrome)

Description

- Leading cause of acquired heart disease in children in the United States
- An acute systemic vasculitis of unknown cause

- Acute, febrile, exanthemous illness
- Seventy-five percent of cases are seen in children less than 5 years (peak age: 18 to 24 months)
- Increased incidence (50% greater) in boys
- Self-limited without treatment; however, 20% of children develop coronary artery dilation or aneurysm
- Infants less than 1 year of age are most seriously affected and at greatest risk of heart involvement
- Often seen in seasonal outbreaks from late winter to early spring

Manifestations

- Kawasaki disease manifests in three phases:
  - Acute phase: Lasts 10 to 14 days
    - Begins with abrupt onset of high fever, unresponsive to antibiotics and antipyretics
  - Subacute phase: Lasts approximately 15 to 25 days
    - Fever disappears
    - Continued irritability and anorexia
    - Desquamation of finger/toes
    - Arthritis, arthralgia
    - Cardiovascular manifestations: Heart failure, dysrhythmias, coronary aneurysms
    - High risk for thrombosis in aneurysm, resulting in myocardial infarction
  - Convalescent phase: Begins on Day 25 and lasts until erythrocyte sedimentation rate returns to normal and all signs of illness have disappeared

FAST FACTS in a NUTSHELL

There have been no firm studies showing a direct link between carpet cleaning and Kawasaki syndrome, although Japanese investigators have proposed an association between house-dust mites and Kawasaki disease. In cases where a child developed Kawasaki syndrome after the carpet was cleaned, it was by a do-it-yourself method or when the child entered the room within 2 hours of cleaning. Therefore, it is best to keep young children (and pets) away from newly cleaned rugs and carpets for at least several hours.

Diagnostic Criteria

- Fever for 5 days or longer with at least four other primary symptoms:
  - Bilateral nonpurulent conjunctivitis
  - Oral mucosal alterations (strawberry tongue, fissured lips, pharyngeal redness)
  - Redness of hand/feet with desquamation
  - Rash on trunk
  - Cervical lymphadenopathy
  - No other known disease process to explain symptoms

Interventions

- Place child in quiet environment (to decrease cardiac workload / irritability)
- Monitor for symptoms of heart failure
- High-dose IV gamma globulin (IVGG) in conjunction with salicylate therapy to decrease prevalence of coronary artery abnormalities (when given within 10 days of fever onset)
- Most children with Kawasaki disease recover fully
- When cardiovascular complications occur, serious morbidity may result

Rheumatic Fever (Rheumatic Heart Disease)

Description

- A systemic, inflammatory, autoimmune disease
- Belongs to a group of disorders known as collagen diseases
- Involves connective tissue: heart, joints, subcutaneous tissues, brain, and blood vessels
- A complication of group A beta-hemolytic streptococcal (GABHS) pharyngitis (manifests 2 to 6 weeks after infection)
- Self-limited illness in school-age children and adolescents

=== *FAST FACTS in a NUTSHELL*

When rheumatic fever is suspected, the nurse should inquire if the child recently experienced a sore throat.

Diagnostic Criteria

- Jones criteria
- Need two major criteria symptoms **or** one major and two minor criteria symptoms for diagnosis.
- Jones criteria is supported with a positive rapid streptococcal antigen test

Jones Criteria (Modified)

Major Criteria:

> Carditis
> Polyarthritis
> Erythema marginatum
> Chorea
> Subcutaneous nodules

Minor Criteria:

> Fever
> Arthralgia
> Previous history of rheumatic fever
> Elevated sedimentation rate
> Leukocytosis
> Altered PR interval on electrocardiogram (ECG)
> Positive C-reactive protein

Interventions

- Goals of medical management:
  - Eradicate hemolytic streptococci infection
  - Prevent permanent cardiac damage
  - Relieve symptoms
  - Prevent recurrence
- Penicillin is the drug of choice (or alternative if penicillin sensitivity)
- Salicylates for inflammation and fever
- Bed rest during acute febrile phase
- Prophylactic use of antibiotics before dental procedures in children with rheumatic fever

CONCLUSION

Understanding the effects of congenital and acquired heart disorders requires knowledge of the hemodynamic process occurring in the structure of the heart. The nurse needs to stay alert, identify early signs of heart failure, and report the findings.

REFERENCES AND FURTHER READING

American Heart Association. (May, 2013). *Children and cholesterol.* Retrieved from http://www.heart.org/HEARTORG/Conditions/Cholesterol/UnderstandYourRiskforHighCholesterol/Children-and-Cholesterol_UCM_305567_Article.jsp

Hockenberry, M., & Wilson, D. (2013). *Wong's essentials of pediatric nursing* (9th ed.). St. Louis, MO: Elsevier.

Leifer, G. (2011). *Introduction to maternity & pediatric nursing* (6th ed.). St. Louis, MO: Elsevier.

Scheinfeld, N. (2013, February). Kawasaki disease. *Medscape.* Retrieved from http://emedicine.medscape.com/article/965367-overview #aw2aab6b2b4

15

Blood and Lymphatic Disorders

The blood and blood-forming organs make up the hematological system. Blood is vital to all body functions. Blood disorders occur when blood components fail to form correctly or when blood values fail to meet normal standards. The components of blood include plasma and the formed elements known as red blood cells, platelets, and white blood cells.

The lymphatic system is a subsystem of the circulatory system. The lymphatic system includes lymphocytes, lymphatic vessels, lymph nodes, the spleen, tonsils, adenoids, and thymus gland. The lymphatic system drains regions of the body to the lymph nodes, where infectious organisms are destroyed and antibody production is stimulated. It returns excess tissue fluid to the blood and defends the body against disease.

Some disorders are specific to the blood or lymphatic system while others affect both systems.

This chapter reviews:

1. Common lymphatic disorders of childhood
2. Common blood disorders found in children
3. Leukemia, which is associated with both lymphatic and blood systems
4. The formula to calculate absolute neutrophil count

COMMON DISORDER OF THE LYMPHATIC SYSTEM

Hodgkin's Disease/Lymphoma

Description

- Neoplastic disease that originates in the lymphic system and primarily involves the lymph nodes
- Can metastasize to other body parts: spleen, liver, bone marrow, lungs
- Rarely seen before 5 years of age
- Incidence increases during adolescence and young adulthood
- Twice as common in boys

Manifestations

- Presenting symptom is a painless lump in the neck or supraclavicular area
- As the disease advances, nonspecific systemic symptoms may include: anorexia, weight loss, night sweats, general malaise, rash, and itching

Diagnostic Criteria

- Chest x-ray or CT of neck and chest
- Positron emission tomography (PET) scan to identify areas of metastatic disease

Staging Hodgkin's Lymphoma

Stage	Criteria
I	Restricted to a single site or group of lymph nodes; asymptomatic
II	Involves two or more lymph nodes in one area or on the same side of the diaphragm
III	Involves lymph node regions on both sides of the diaphragm; involves adjacent organs or spleen
IV	Is diffuse; least favorable prognosis

- Blood tests: complete blood count, erythrocyte sedimentation rate, serum copper, ferritin level, fibrinogen, uric acid level immunoglobulins, liver function tests, T-cell function studies, and urinalysis
- Lymph node biopsy for diagnosis and staging, with presence of giant multinucleated cells called Reed-Sternberg cells

Interventions

- Both radiation therapy and chemotherapy are used in accordance with the clinical stage of the disease
- COPP regime is the protocol; that is, a combination of cyclophosphamide and vincristine (Oncovin), procarbazine hydrochloride, and prednisone
- Nursing care is directed toward symptomatic relief of radiation and chemotherapy side effects including hair loss, impaired immunity, nausea, mouth sores, and skin irritation
- Long-term prognosis is excellent

═══════════════════════════════*FAST FACTS in a NUTSHELL*

A risk factor that should be discussed prior to treatment with radiation and chemotherapy is the high risk of sterility from treatment. Sperm banking is now offered at many cancer centers.

COMMON DISORDERS OF THE BLOOD SYSTEM

Leukemia

Description

- A group of malignant diseases of the blood-forming tissues; that is, the bone marrow and lymphatic system
- Two forms are generally found in children:
  - Acute lymphoid leukemia (ALL)
  - Acute nonlymphoid (myelogenous) leukemia (ANLL or AML)
- Most common form of childhood cancer
- Peak onset between 2 and 5 years of age
- More common in boys

Manifestations

- Low-grade fever
- Pallor, bruising, and leg and joint pain
- Listlessness, abdominal pain
- Enlarged lymph nodes, liver, or spleen

FAST FACTS in a NUTSHELL

Active routine immunizations against live viral vaccines such as measles, mumps, and rubella are delayed while the child is receiving immunosuppressive drugs. Most institutions have guidelines for vaccinations in children undergoing immunosuppressive therapy.

Diagnostic Criteria

- History and symptoms
- Bone marrow aspiration provides definitive diagnosis
  - Decreased red blood cells (RBCs), platelets, and normal white blood cells (WBCs), but overproduction of immature WBCs or blasts

Interventions

- Use of chemotherapeutic agents in four phases
  - Induction therapy
  - Central nervous system prophylactic therapy
  - Intensification therapy
  - Maintenance therapy
- Hematopoietic stem cell transplantation has been used successfully but is not the initial treatment for ALL
- Prevent infection secondary to neutropenia
- Prognosis continues to improve and long-term survival is dependent on initial WBC count, age, type of cell involved, sex of the child, and karyotype analysis
- Child may return to school when absolute neutrophil count is greater than 500/mm

Calculating Absolute Neutrophil Count

Determine the total percent of neutrophils (includes neutrophils and nonsegmented neutrophils such as bands).

Multiply WBC count by percentage of neutrophils.

Example:

WBC = 1,000 neutrophils = 7% nonsegmented neutrophils = 7%

Step 1: 7% + 7% = 14%

Step 2: $0.14 \times 1,000 = 140$ absolute neutrophil count (ANC)

Hemophilia

Description

- Group of bleeding disorders in which there is a defect in the clotting mechanism
- X-linked recessive trait in most cases (alternating generations)
- The two most common types:
  - Hemophilia A (deficiency in factor VIII or AHG antihemophilic globulin); also called *classic hemophilia*. Hemophilia A accounts for the majority of cases.
  - Hemophila B (factor IX deficiency); also called *Christmas disease*.

Manifestations

- Usually not apparent in the newborn unless excess bleeding occurs at the umbilical cord or after circumcision
- As child grows and becomes more active, clinical symptoms may include:
  - Prolonged bleeding anywhere (blood clotting requires 1 hour or longer)
  - Hemorrhage from any trauma
  - Excessive bruising

- Subcutaneous and intramuscular hemorrhages
- Hemarthrosis (especially the knees, ankles, and elbows)
- Hematomas
- Spontaneous hematuria
• Anemia

FAST FACTS in a NUTSHELL

> When bleeding occurs in a child with hemophilia, the best action to take is rest, ice, compression, and elevation (RICE).

Diagnostic Criteria

• History and symptoms presented
• Partial thromboplastin time (PTT)
• Specific factor deficiencies
• Prenatal diagnosis by amniocentesis for carrier detection in classic hemophilia

Interventions

• Prevent bleeding by replacing the missing factor
• Treatment: Factor VIII concentrate from genetically engineered recombinant or pooled plasma (infusions given three times a week)
• Synthetic form of vasopressin increases plasma factor VIII activity
• Avoid contact sports
• Encourage normal life and appropriate activities

Iron-Deficiency Anemia

Anemia refers to a condition in which the number or size of RBCs or the hemoglobin (Hgb) concentration is below normal values for age. This diminishes the oxygen-carrying capacity of the blood, causing a reduction in the oxygen available to the tissues. Anemia is a common blood disorder of childhood and is not a disease but an indication of an underlying pathologic process. Iron-deficiency anemia is specific to insufficient amounts of iron in the body.

Incidence

- The most common nutritional deficiency in the United States
- May be caused by insufficient intake of iron in the diet, inability to absorb iron, or severe hemorrhage
- Good prenatal diet by the mother can provide adequate stores for the full-term infant to last 5 to 6 months
- Low birth-weight infants and/or multiple births can result in low stores of iron

Manifestations

- Pallor, irritability
- Anorexia, decreased activity
- Heart murmur may be present
- Enlarged spleen

FAST FACTS in a NUTSHELL

Question: What method should be used to give oral iron supplements to a child?

Answer: Milk and milk products interfere with iron absorption so they should be avoided. Since vitamin C aids in the absorption of iron; it is ideal to give a vitamin C supplement between meals with juice. Liquid iron preparations can stain the teeth and should be taken through a straw.

Diagnostic Criteria

- RBC count including mean corpuscular volume (MCV)
  - Infants MCV below 70 mcm^3 is diagnostic
  - MCV 70 mcm^3 plus child's age in years = lower limit of normal for children ages 1 to 10 years
- Dietary history of child (prenatal history if infant)

Interventions

- Ferrous sulfate given orally 2 to 3 times a day between meals
- Vitamin C helps in the absorption of iron
- Foods high in iron are added to the diet

- Iron-fortified formula during first year (if not breastfeeding)
- Solid foods high in iron are encouraged as age appropriate: egg yolk, leafy green vegetables, dried fruits, whole grains, iron-fortified cereals

Sickle Cell Anemia/Sickle Cell Disease

Includes *all* hereditary disorders in which the clinical, hematologic, and pathologic features are related to the presence of hemoglobin (Hgb) that is partly or completely replaced by abnormal sickle Hgb (HbS).

Description

- Sickle cell anemia is one of a group of diseases in which normal adult Hgb (Hgb A) is partly or completely replaced by abnormal sickle Hgb (HbS)
- Of sickle cell disease, sickle cell anemia is the most common form in African Americans and one of the most common genetic diseases worldwide
- Autosomal recessive disorder or inherited defect in the formation of hemoglobin
- These cells are fragile and have difficulty passing through capillaries, causing "pile up" in small vessels
- Two types:
  - Sickle cell trait: Presence of both normal Hgb A and abnormal HbS but asymptomatic. Inherited from one parent.
  - Sickle cell anemia: Inherited from both parents. Each offspring has a 1:4 chance of inheriting the disease.

Manifestations

- General symptoms: Growth retardation and/or delay in sexual maturation, chronic anemia (Hgb 6–9 g/dL), and susceptibility to infection
- Pale, tires easily, little appetite
- Symptoms appear at the end of infancy or during toddler or preschool years
- *Sickle cell crisis*: Acutely ill due to exacerbation of the condition
  - Vaso-occlusion with pain in the area of involvement:
    - Painful swelling of hands and feet, muscle spasms, and swollen joints

- Abdominal pain, fever, and vomiting
- Hematuria, jaundice, and hepatic coma
- Stroke, visual disturbances, convulsions, and paralysis
- Chest syndrome resembling pneumonia and pulmonary disease
- Sickle cells block microcirculation, causing pooling of large amounts of blood resulting in hepatomegaly, splenomegaly, and circulatory collapse
- Chronic vaso-occlusive phenomena result over time

Diagnostic Criteria

- Before birth, chorionic villi sampling can detect disease
- Newborn screening for sickle cell anemia (Sickledex) is mandatory in most states
- Hemoglobin electrophoresis distinguishes between sickle cell trait and sickle cell anemia

Interventions

- Provide supportive, symptomatic treatment and prevent sickle cell crisis
  - Blood transfusions (erythrocytapheresis) to replace sickle cells with normal RBCs
  - Analgesics
  - Fluid/electrolyte control
  - Prevention of infection
- Splenectomy in recurrent splenic sequestration
- Pneumococcal and meningococcal vaccines
- Prognosis varies, most live into fifth decade
- Hematopoietic stem cell transplantation offers a curative approach for some children with sickle cell disease

=====*FAST FACTS in a NUTSHELL*

Meperidine (Demerol) is contraindicated for use in managing the pain associated with sickle cell crisis.

Normeperidine is a metabolite of Demerol and a central nervous system stimulant. Patients with sickle cell disease are particularly at risk for normeperidine-induced seizures.

Thalassemia/Beta-Thalassemia/Thalassemia Major/Cooley Anemia

Description

- A group of inherited disorders characterized by an abnormal hemoglobin synthesis that results from a reduction in or absence of one of the chains found in normal hemoglobin
- The RBCs are abnormal in size and shape and are rapidly destroyed
- Inherited, autosomal recessive pattern. If the child inherits only one gene, may exhibit only mild anemia (thalassemia minor)
- Highest incidence (gene carriers) are those of Italian, Greek, and Syrian ancestry
- Beta-thalassemia is the most common of the thalassemias
- Two forms of beta-thalassemia
  - Thalassemia minor: Trait inherited from one parent resulting in mild anemia, pale appearance. Often misdiagnosed with iron-deficiency anemia
  - Thalassemia major (Cooley's anemia): Two thalassemia genes inherited and result in a more serious form of the disease
- RBCs are abnormal in size and shape and are rapidly destroyed, which results in anemia
- To compensate for hemolytic process, an overabundance of erythrocytes are formed

Manifestations

- Impairs erythrocyte's ability to carry O_2; can result in hypoxia
- Severe anemia: Pallor, fever, poor appetite, and enlarged spleen and liver resulting in great abdominal distention and organ pressure
- Growth and maturation retardation
- Bronze skin tone
- Bone changes: characteristic enlarged head, frontal and parietal bossing, severe maxillary hyperplasia, malocclusion
- Cardiac failure is a threat

Diagnostic Criteria

- Family history

Question: What causes the bronzed complexion in children with thalassemia major?

Answer: The muddy bronze color results from hemosiderosis, a deposit of iron into the tissues as a result of rapid destruction of blood cells.

- Radiographic bone growth studies
- CBC with low Hgb count
- Hgb electrophoresis confirms the diagnosis

Interventions

- To maintain sufficient Hgb levels to prevent bone marrow expansion and support normal growth and development
- Blood transfusions
- Chelation therapy to minimize hemosiderosis
- Splenectomy may be necessary
- Hematopoietic stem cell transplantation is a curative treatment for some children
- With early intervention, most children will survive well into adulthood

CONCLUSION

Since the major blood-forming organs of the body are the red bone marrow and lymphatic system, disorders affecting these organs often result in RBC, WBC, or platelet disorders reflected in symptoms of bleeding, infection, and/or altered tissue oxygenation.

REFERENCES AND FURTHER READING

Determining your ANC (absolute neutrophil count). (n.d.). Retrieved from http://depts.washington.edu/registry/Calculate.ANC.pdf

Hockenberry, M., & Wilson, D. (2013). *Wong's essentials of pediatric nursing* (9th ed.). St. Louis, MO: Elsevier.

Leifer, G. (2011). *Introduction to maternity & pediatric nursing* (6th ed.). St. Louis, MO: Elsevier.

16

Gastrointestinal Disorders:
Dysfunctional, Structural,
and Obstructive Disorders

There are distinct differences between the child and adult in regard to the gastrointestinal (GI) system. The newborn has a decreased resistance to bacterial and viral infections due to incomplete development of the GI system. Due to greater percentage of total body water, children will experience dehydration more quickly than adults if nausea, vomiting, and/or diarrhea occur. The hepatic efficiency of the newborn is immature and can cause jaundice. Some congenital defects of the GI system are not evident at birth and may result in a compromise in growth due to delayed diagnosis. The pediatric nurse should be alert to identifying changes in diet and elimination in children. Early recognition and treatment of GI disorders can prevent the child from falling behind in expected growth and development.

This chapter reviews:

1. Common GI dysfunctions
2. Congenital structural defects
3. Common obstructive disorders in children

GI DYSFUNCTION

GI disorders in this group have the greatest potential for causing serious alterations in fluid and electrolyte balance. Most of the diagnoses found in this category are directly related to disorders of motility, inflammation, infection, or infestation.

GI dysfunctions are often caused by infectious agents in the GI tract, whereas noninfectious causes of diarrhea involve food intolerance, overfeeding, improper formula preparation, or ingestion of high amounts of a sugar-free additive (sorbitol).

Vomiting

Description

- Forceful ejection of gastric contents through the mouth
- Common symptom during infancy/childhood and usually self-limiting

Manifestations

- May be associated with other processes, such as infectious disease, increased intracranial pressure, toxic ingestion, food intolerance, mechanical obstruction, metabolic disorders, and psychological stress

Diagnostic Criteria

- Accurate assessment of type and appearance of vomitus
- Assessment of the child's behavior in association with vomiting helps to establish a diagnosis

Interventions

- Nursing interventions directed to identifying and treating the cause
- Assess fluid and electrolyte status
- Position to prevent aspiration

Description

- Gastroenteritis is the leading cause of illness in children younger than 5 years of age
- Rotavirus is the most important cause of serious gastroenteritis for children in developed nations
- Other infectious agents such as viruses, bacteria, and parasites can be a cause of gastroenteritis in children throughout the world

Manifestations

- Sudden increase in frequency and a change in consistency of stools
- May be associated with upper respiratory infections, urinary tract infections, or antibiotic therapy
- Usually self-limiting, will resolve if dehydration does not occur
- Dehydration
- Acid—base imbalance
- Shock

FAST FACTS in a NUTSHELL

Question: At what age is the rotavirus vaccine no longer an option for prevention of rotavirus?

Answer: The rotavirus vaccine is usually given at 2 and 4 months of age. The maximum age for the final dose in the series is 8 months, 0 days.

Diagnostic Criteria

- History of presenting symptoms and any recent travel, change in diet, contact with animals, and daycare center attendance
- An enzyme-linked immunosorbent assay (ELISA) may confirm rotavirus or *Giardia* organisms
- *Clostridium difficile* toxin may be found with recent antibiotic history

Interventions

- Assess fluid and electrolyte balance
  - Weigh daily
- Rehydrate; oral rehydration therapy (ORT) should be used first
- Maintain fluid therapy
- Reintroduce diet
- Prevent excoriation of skin to perineum

Constipation

Description

- Defecation that is infrequent or difficulty in passing hard, dry stool

Manifestations

- Frequency of bowel movements can vary widely in children; not considered diagnostic criteria
- Long periods of constipation can result in encopresis or fecal soiling

Diagnostic Criteria

- Constipation can be a symptom of an environmental, psychosocial, or disorder outside the GI tract

Interventions

- Evaluate dietary and bowel habits
- Promote regular bowel movements (same time of day)
- Add fiber and/or fluids to daily routine

Hirschsprung Disease

Description

- A congenital anomaly; occurs when there is an absence of ganglionic innervation to the muscle of a segment of the bowel (usually in the lower sigmoid colon)
- Four times more common in males and follows a familial pattern

Manifestations

- Failure to pass meconium stool in newborn
- Abdominal distention, megacolon, anorexia, failure to thrive
- Chronic constipation with episodes of diarrhea and vomiting
- Ribbon-like, foul-smelling stools

Diagnostic Criteria

- Barium enema and rectal biopsy

Interventions

- Impaired portion of colon is removed with anastomosis
- Temporary colostomy may be necessary

Gastroesophageal Reflux (GER)

Description

- Transfer of gastric contents into the esophagus as a result of incompetent or relaxed lower esophageal sphincter (LES)
- Associated with neuromuscular delay

Manifestations

- Often seen in preterm infants and children with neuromuscular disorders
- Vomiting within first and second weeks of life
- Fussy and hungry
- Respiratory problems (apnea) can occur when vomiting stimulates the closure of epiglottis

═══════════════════════ *FAST FACTS in a NUTSHELL*

Question: Should GER always be treated in infants?

Answer: Approximately 50% of all infants younger than 2 months are reported to have GER. No therapy is needed if the infant is thriving and no respiratory complications are present. The symptoms of GER usually decrease around 12 months of age, when the infant is more upright. The physician needs to differentiate between GER and GERD.

16. GASTROINTESTINAL DISORDERS: DYSFUNCTIONAL, STRUCTURAL, AND OBSTRUCTIVE DISORDERS

Diagnostic Criteria

- History of symptoms and physical exam
- Upper GI series to evaluate anatomic abnormalities
- 24-hour intraesophageal pH monitoring study is the gold standard in diagnosis
- Endoscopy with biopsy may help to exclude other disorders

Interventions

- Thickened feeding (1 teaspoon to 1 tablespoon of rice cereal per ounce of formula)
- Careful burping, avoid overfeeding, place upright after feeding
- Pharmacologic therapy (H_2-receptor antagonists and proton pump inhibitors) may be used to treat infants and children with GERD that has resulted from GER

Appendicitis

Description

- Inflammation of the vermiform appendix (blind sac at end of the cecum)
- Small appendage becomes obstructed by infection, fecal material, parasites, and so forth
- Most common reason for emergency abdominal surgery in childhood
- Average age of onset is 10 years

Manifestations

- Periumbilical pain localizes to right lower quadrant, nausea, and later vomiting
- Guarding (rigidity of abdomen on palpation)
- Rebound tenderness

Diagnostic Criteria

- On exam, characteristic tenderness at McBurney's point in right lower quadrant of abdomen
- Elevation of white blood cells (neutrophils increased by 75% with perforation)
- X-ray of kidneys/ureter/bladder will reveal dilated cecum

- Nothing by mouth (NPO) status
- Assess for signs of perforation

══════════════════════════════*FAST FACTS in a NUTSHELL*

If the child being evaluated for appendicitis reports a sudden relief of acute pain, suspect perforation of the appendix! The nurse should assess for signs of peritonitis (rigid guarding, abdominal distention, tachycardia, and chills), notify the physician, and anticipate the need for emergency surgery.

Thrush (Oral Candidiasis)

Description

- Infection of the mucous membranes caused by the fungus *Candida.*

Manifestations

- White patches that resemble milk curds appear on the oral mucosa
- Anorexia
- Can pass to esophagus, stomach, and diaper area

Diagnostic Criteria

- Presenting symptoms as listed above

Interventions

- Antifungal suspension such as mycostatin (Nystatin) 3 to 4 times daily
- Antifungal creams (Nystatin) can also be used to treat diaper rash

Worms/Enterobiasis/Pinworms

Description

- The most common variety of worm that affects children
- Appears as a white thread about 1/3-inch long
- Route of entry is mouth
- Lives in lower intestine but comes out of the anus to deposit eggs during the night

Manifestations

- Itching and scratching around anal area
- Irritability, fretfulness at night
- Poor appetite, weight loss

Diagnostic Criteria

- Tape test to obtain eggs (done in early morning)

Interventions

- Anthelmintics, such as Pyrantel
- Treat all symptomatic members of the family to prevent reinfection

Worms/Ascariasis/Roundworms

Description

- Roundworm infestation more commonly seen in southern states
- Eggs from infected person can survive in the soil and be ingested by a child

Manifestations

- Asymptomatic or causes abdominal pain
- Chronic cough without fever is characteristic

- Eggs develop into larvae in the intestine and can penetrate to the liver and circulate to lungs and heart
- When larvae reach glottis, they are coughed up and swallowed to small intestines where they develop and grow

Diagnostic Criteria

- Stool specimen positive for presence of ova and/or parasite

Interventions

- Anthelmintics, such as albendazole

STRUCTURAL DEFECTS

The GI disorders in this group are related to a defect or malformation that has occurred somewhere along the GI tract. Structural defects are a result of interruption or failure of cellular processes during embryonic development. Some congenital malformations are easily identifiable at birth, while others may not be initially as apparent.

Cleft Lip

Description

- A fissure or opening in the upper lip as a result of failure of the maxillary and median nasal processes to unite during the 4th through 10th week of development
- The most common congenital deformity in the United States
- Hereditary predisposition or can be caused by environmental teratogens
- More common in boys

Manifestations

- Incomplete closure of the lip. Can be slight to severe, unilateral or bilateral

FAST FACTS in a NUTSHELL

Question: In an infant with both cleft lip and cleft palate, which surgical repair will be completed first, and why?

Answer: The lip is repaired first not only to improve sucking but also to improve appearance and facilitate infant/parent bonding.

Diagnostic Criteria

• Evident at birth

Interventions

• Surgical repair (*cheiloplasty*)
• "Rule of 10s": Child is 10 weeks of age, weighs 10 pounds, and hemoglobin of 10
• Excellent prognosis with minimal scarring

Cleft Palate

Description

• Failure of the hard palate to fuse at the midline during gestational development
• Forms a passageway between the nasopharynx and nose

Manifestations

• May not be readily apparent at birth
• Unable to create suction in the oral cavity necessary for feeding

Diagnostic Criteria

• Visual examination of the oral cavity or found on palpation with gloved finger

Interventions

- Use of special needs feeder until surgical repair
- Cleft palate surgical repair typically occurs between 6 and 12 months of age. Earlier repair may interfere with skeletal growth of the mid-face. Later repair can interfere with speech development

Esophageal Atresia (Tracheoesophageal Fistula; TEF)

Description

- Caused by a failure of the tissues of the GI tract to separate properly from the respiratory tract early in prenatal life
- Four variations of this disorder are differentiated by the esophagus connections (esophageal atresia is the most common variation)

Manifestations

- Earliest sign of TEF occurs prenatally when the mother develops polyhydramnios (the fetus is unable to swallow amniotic fluid, resulting in accumulation of fluid in the sac)
- Drooling or frothy mucus from nose or mouth
- Apnea or vomiting with first feeding
- Abdominal distention

Diagnostic Criteria

- Radiographic studies

=======*FAST FACTS in a NUTSHELL*

The three "Cs" used in the clinical diagnosis of TEF are: coughing, choking, and cyanosis (noted with first feeding).

Interventions

- Maintain patent airway and prevent pneumonia; keep NPO, suction airway as needed, position to drain mucus from the nose and throat
- Surgical repair of the anomaly

Hernia

Description

- A protrusion of a portion of an organ through an abnormal opening or defect
- Umbilical hernia is a protrusion of a portion of the intestine through the umbilical ring
- Inguinal hernia is a protrusion of part of the abdominal contents through the inguinal canal. More common in preterm males

Manifestations

- A mass appears, especially when the child cries or strains
- Reducible—can be put back in place with gentle pressure
- Irreducible or incarcerated—unable to put back in place
- Strangulated—when intestine is caught and blood supply is diminished

Diagnostic Criteria

- Physical exam with palpable mass

Interventions

- Surgical repair: herniorrhaphy

FAST FACTS in a NUTSHELL

Following a herniorrhaphy, one of the most significant assessment findings is the return of bowel function.

Obstruction in the GI tract occurs when the passage of nutrients and secretions is impeded by occlusion, stricture, or impaired motility. Obstructions may be congenital and be readily apparent during the neonatal period or appear after a few weeks of life. Other obstructions can be acquired during infancy or childhood.

Hypertrophic Pyloric Stenosis (HPS)

Description

- A narrowing or stenosis of the lower end of the stomach, caused by overgrowth of circular muscles of the pylorus or by spasms of the sphincter
- Usually develops in the first few weeks of life (rarely after 2 months)

Manifestations

- Projectile vomiting immediately after feeding
- Growth failure, dehydration, depressed fontanelles, and chronic hunger
- Olive-shaped mass in right upper quadrant of the abdomen
- Peristaltic waves are visible during feeding

FAST FACTS in a NUTSHELL

There is a heredity tendency in HPS. This disorder is more likely in first-born males.

Diagnostic Criteria

- History of presenting symptoms and physical exam (see above)
- Ultrasonography

Interventions

- Surgical repair: pyloromyotomy as soon as possible, if not dehydrated

Intussusception

Description

- One segment of the bowel telescopes into another segment, pulling mesentery with it
- Most common site is the ileocecal valve
- Intussusception is the most common cause of intestinal obstruction in children between the ages of 3 months and 3 years
- More common in boys and in children with cystic fibrosis
- Cause is unknown

Manifestations

- Classic triad of symptoms: abdominal pain, abdominal mass, bloody stools
- Drawing of knees into the chest
- Currant jelly-like stools
- Fever and shock can occur

Diagnostic Criteria

- Ultrasonography

Interventions

- Considered an emergency
- Conservative treatment via air, saline, or barium enema (10% of cases corrected)
- Laparoscopic surgical repair if conservative treatment not effective

Imperforate Anus/Anal Rectal Malformations

Description

- Failure of separation between the two tissues that allow for a passageway between the lower GI tract and the anus
- The lower end of the GI tract and the anus end in blind pouches
- Range from stenosis to complete separation or failure of the anus to form

Manifestations

- Absence of external opening or failure for insertion of rectal probe upon birth
- Failure to pass meconium stool during first 24 hours after birth
- Meconium presence in urine
- Abdominal distention

Diagnostic Criteria

- Physical exam revealing absent anus or blind pouch in passageway
- Abdominal and pelvic ultrasonography, magnetic resonance imaging (MRI)

Interventions

- Surgical or laparoscopic repair, anoplasty, or colostomy

═══════════════════════════════════*FAST FACTS in a NUTSHELL*

Since many GI disorders result in vague symptoms, encouraging the parent to keep a detailed diary or written account of symptoms may be helpful in reaching a timely diagnosis.

REFERENCES AND FURTHER READING

Centers for Disease Control and Prevention. (n.d.). *Facts about cleft lip and cleft palate.* Retrieved from http://www.cdc.gov/ncbddd/birthdefects/cleftlip.html

Hockenberry, M., & Wilson, D. (2013). *Wong's essentials of pediatric nursing* (9th ed.). St. Louis, MO: Elsevier.

Leifer, G. (2011). *Introduction to maternity & pediatric nursing* (6th ed.). St. Louis, MO: Elsevier.

17

Gastrointestinal Disorders: Malabsorption Syndromes, Nutritional Deficiencies, and Poisoning

The extensive area of the gastrointestinal (GI) tract not only provides a greater exchange between the child and the environment, but also a greater chance for GI problems to surface. The significant difference between the child and adult is the increased need for nutrition. The infant has a small stomach that empties rapidly, and thus requires more frequent feedings. The child grows continuously but also enters growth spurts. The nutritional, metabolic, and energy needs increase during growth. The infant has a limited ability to absorb fat because of decreased bile acid; therefore, unlike adults, the infant requires more fat in the daily diet. Children are curious explorers and are at greater risk for accidental poisoning. The pediatric nurse must know normal growth and development so as to identify when nutritional deficiencies occur. The pediatric nurse is a teacher, child advocate, and preventive health care provider.

This chapter reviews:

1. Childhood malabsorption syndromes
2. Nutritional deficiencies in children
3. Poisonings common among children

MALABSORPTION SYNDROMES

Chronic diarrhea and malabsorption of nutrients characterize malabsorption syndromes. The consequence can result in growth failure in children. The exact cause is unknown but is believed to be an inherited cell-mediated immunologic overstimulation.

Celiac Disease (Gluten-Sensitive Enteropathy)

Description

- A permanent intestinal intolerance to dietary wheat gluten and related proteins that produces mucosal lesions in genetically susceptible individuals
- More frequent in children of European descent

Manifestations

- Failure to thrive, irritable
- Stools are large, bulky, and frothy
- Enlarged abdomen and atrophy of buttocks

Diagnostic Criteria

- Diagnosis confirmed with serum immunoglobin A (IgA) test and small bowel biopsy
- On biopsy of the small intestine, finding villous atrophy with hyperplasia of the crypts and abnormal epithelium in a child eating gluten

Interventions

- Lifelong diet restriction of wheat, barley, oats, and rye

NUTRITIONAL DEFICIENCIES

Adequate nutrients are essential during times of growth. The most rapid periods of growth in children occur during infancy and adolescence. Although severe malnutrition and vitamin deficiencies are more commonly found in developing countries, poverty or neglect or lack of knowledge can contribute to nutritional deficits anywhere in the world.

Failure to Thrive (FTT)

Description

- Infants and children who fail to gain and often lose weight without an obvious cause
- Can be associated with pathological dysfunction (such as heart disease or malabsorption), lack of parent–infant bonding, or result from environmental stressors or factors

Manifestations

- Child falls below the third percentile in weight and height on a standard growth chart
- Development is delayed
- Hypotonia, irritable, pica (eating nonfood items)

Diagnostic Criteria

- History of presenting symptoms and physical exam revealing delayed physical development

Interventions

- Provide sufficient calories to support catch-up growth
- Treat any medical causes for malabsorption
- Multidisciplinary approach and support to child and family

Protein Deficiency/Kwashiorkor

Description

- Severe protein deficiency despite adequate calorie intake

Manifestations

- Usually occurs in children ages 1 to 4 years (after removal from the breast)
- Edema to the abdomen; muscles are weak and wasted
- Diarrhea, skin infections, irritability, anorexia, and vomiting
- Growth retardation
- Depigmentation (white streak in the hair) due to melanin deficit

Diagnostic Criteria

- History and physical exam for symptoms (see above)

Interventions

- Preventive treatment with education and support to the family
- Protein-rich diet

Vitamin D Deficiency/Rickets

Description

- Deficiency of vitamin D resulting in demineralization of bone
- Exposure to sunlight and vitamin D are necessary for metabolism of calcium and phosphorus, which are needed for normal bone growth

Manifestations

- Bowlegs, knock-knees, beading of ribs called *rachitic rosary*
- Improper teeth formation

Diagnostic Criteria

- History and physical exam

Interventions

- Vitamin D, vitamin D-fortified milk, and well-balanced meals
- Exposure to outdoor sunlight

Vitamin C Deficiency/Scurvy

Description

- Insufficient intake or absorption of vitamin C

Manifestations

- Joint pain
- Bleeding gums and loose teeth
- Lack of energy

- History and physical exam

Interventions

- Vitamin C added to diet; good food sources of vitamin C include citrus fruits, raw leafy vegetables
- Vitamin C is water soluble so is not stored by the body

═══════════════════════════════════*FAST FACTS in a NUTSHELL*

> When encountering vitamin C deficiency in children, the nurse needs to assess the method by which food is prepared. Vitamin C is easily destroyed by heat and exposure to air.

INGESTION OF HARMFUL SUBSTANCES/ POISONING

Poisoning in children, especially before the age of 6 years, continues to be a health concern in pediatric nursing. Although pharmaceuticals such as analgesics, cold preparations, topical preparations, antibiotics, vitamins, hormones, and antihistamines are agents involved in poisoning, the most common substances involved in poisoning of children are included in this section. Children are curious explorers and can be exposed to toxic substances, which are readily accessible in the home environment.

═══════════════════════════════════*FAST FACTS in a NUTSHELL*

> Ingestion of harmful substances should be treated as an emergency.
>
> 1. Assess the child and initiate ABCs (airway, breathing, circulation) as appropriate.
> 2. Terminate exposure.
> 3. Identify the poison.
> 4. Contact Poison Control Center.
>
> **In the United States (Voice/TTY): 1-800-222-1222**
>
> 5. Prevent poison absorption.

Corrosive Substances (Strong Acids and Alkali)

Description

- Drain, toilet, and oven cleaners; dishwasher detergents; mildew remover; batteries; denture cleaners; bleach
- Liquid corrosives cause more damage than granular preparations

Manifestations

- Severe burning in the mouth, throat, and stomach
- White, swollen mucous membranes
- Edema of lips, tongue, and pharynx; can result in respiratory obstruction
- Violent vomiting
- Drooling and inability to clear secretions
- Signs of shock, anxiety, and agitation

Diagnostic Criteria

- Evidence or suspicion of ingestion

Interventions

- Contact the poison control center (PCC) immediately
- Do NOT induce vomiting
- Maintain patent airway
- No oral intake (unless instructed by PCC)
- Esophageal strictures may require repeated dilatation

Hydrocarbon Ingestion

Description

- Gasoline, kerosene, mineral oil, paint thinner, turpentine, lighter fluid
- Immediate danger is aspiration and pneumonia

Manifestations

- Gagging, choking, coughing
- Nausea, vomiting

- Lethargy, weakness
- Respiratory symptoms (tachypnea, cyanosis, retractions, grunting)

Diagnostic Criteria

- Evidence or suspecion of ingestion

Interventions

- Do NOT induce vomiting
- Treatment is directed toward symptoms of chemical pneumonia (high-humidity oxygen, hydration, and antibiotics to prevent secondary infection)

Acetaminophen (Tylenol) Poisoning

Description

- Overdose or overingestion of Tylenol
- Toxic dose is 150 mg/kg or greater
- Most common accidental drug poisoning in children

Manifestations

- Occurs in four stages:
  - Initial (2 to 4 hours after ingestion)
    - Nausea, vomiting, sweating, pallor
  - Latent period (24 to 36 hours after ingestion)
    - Improvement of symptoms
  - Hepatic involvement
    - Right upper quadrant pain
    - Jaundice, confusion, stupor, coagulation problems
  - Recovery or death

Diagnostic Criteria

- Evidence or suspicion of ingestion

Interventions

- Antidote N-acetylcysteine given orally (may mix in juice to counter odor); given as loading dose then followed with maintenance doses

Acetylsalicylic Acid (Aspirin) Poisoning

Description

- May be caused by acute ingestion (300 to 500 mg/kg)
- Chronic ingestion (more than 100 mg/kg/day for 2 or more days)

Manifestations

- Nausea, vomiting, dehydration, oliguria
- Disorientation, diaphoresis
- Hyperpnea, tinnitus
- Hyperpyrexia, coma, convulsions

Diagnostic Criteria

- Evidence or suspicion of ingestion

Interventions

- Induce vomiting, gastric lavage, or administer activated charcoal and/or cathartics
- Sodium bicarbonate transfusion to correct metabolic acidosis
- Anticonvulsants, use external cooling for hyperpyrexia
- Administer vitamin K for bleeding
- Oxygen and ventilation as needed
- Hemodialysis in severe cases

Poisonous Plants

Description

- Plants are some of the most frequently ingested substances
- Rarely cause serious problems (sometimes fatal)

Manifestations

- Depends on plant ingested (see Table 17.1 for list of poisonous plants and toxic parts)
- May cause local irritation of oropharynx and entire GI tract
- May cause choking and allergic reactions
- May cause respiratory, renal, and central nervous system symptoms
- Topical contact can result in dermatitis

TABLE 17.1 Poisonous Plants and Toxic Parts

Apple (leaves, seeds)	Mistletoe (berries, leaves)
Apricot (leaves, stem, seeds)	Oak tree (acorn, foliage)
Azalea (all parts)	Philodendron (all parts)
Buttercup (all parts)	Plum (pit)
Castor (bean or seeds extremely toxic)	Poinsettia (leaves)
Cherry (twigs, seeds, foliage)	Poison ivy, poison oak (leaves, stem, sap, fruit, smoke from burning plant)
Daffodil (bulbs)	Pokeweed, pokeberry (roots, berries, leaves)
Dumbcane—Dieffenbachia (all parts)	Pothos (all parts)
Elephant ear (all parts)	Rhubarb (leaves)
English ivy (all parts)	Tulip (bulbs)
Foxglove (leaves, seeds, flowers)	Water hemlock (all parts)
Holly (berries, leaves)	Wisteria (seeds, pods)
Hyacinth (bulbs)	Yew (all parts)

Avoid using these plants in or around the home where young children reside.

Diagnostic Criteria

- Evidence or suspicion of ingestion

Interventions

- Induce vomiting
- Wash skin and eyes
- Provide supportive care

Lead Poisoning (Plumbism)

Description

- Repeated absorption, inhalation, or ingestion of substances that contain lead
- Increased incidence seen in toddlers
- Being exposed to lead during pregnancy can lead to problems in the newborn

Common sources of lead include paint manufactured before 1978, lead crystal, battery casings, some ceramics, lead curtain weights, fishing sinkers, lead solder, and toys and jewelry made in other countries.

Manifestations

- Early signs: weakness, weight loss, anorexia, pallor, irritability, vomiting, abdominal pain, and constipation
- Later signs: anemia, nervous system involvement (muscular incoordination, neuritis, convulsions, encephalitis)
- Chronic lead toxicity may affect physical growth and reproductive ability

Diagnostic Criteria

- Venous lead level of 5 mcg/dL or higher
- Screening at age 1 or 2 years
- X-ray of the bones
- History of pica eating

Interventions

- Prevention is key
  - Determine source and remove child from lead-hazardous environment/source
  - Read all labels on toys manufactured outside the United States
- Chelation therapy to render the lead nontoxic and increase excretion in the urine

REFERENCES AND FURTHER READING

Centers for Disease Control and Prevention. (n.d.). *Facts about cleft lip and cleft palate.* Retrieved from http://www.cdc.gov/ncbddd/birthdefects/cleftlip.html

Hockenberry, M., & Wilson, D. (2013). *Wong's essentials of pediatric nursing* (9th ed.). St. Louis, MO: Elsevier.

Leifer, G. (2011). *Introduction to maternity & pediatric nursing* (6th ed.). St. Louis, MO: Elsevier.

18

Genitourinary Disorders

Incidence and type of kidney and urinary tract dysfunctions change with age and the presenting complaints can vary with maturation of the child. According to the American Society of Pediatric Nephrology (ASPN), each year in the United States:

- *1,200,000 children develop urinary tract infections (UTIs).*
- *300,000 children will develop disorders that cause blood and protein to leak into their urine, such as glomerulonephritis.*
- *20,000 children are born with kidney abnormalities.*

This chapter reviews:

1. Common genitourinary tract disorders and defects
2. Glomerular disease in children
3. Wilm's tumor description and management

GENITOURINARY TRACT DISORDERS AND DEFECTS

Genitourinary dysfunction is a category associated with either infection along the urinary tract or an external congenital defect. This group of disorders presents as the most common conditions found in childhood.

Urinary Tract Infection

A variety of organisms can be responsible for infections in the urinary tract. *Escherichia coli* (*E. coli*) and other gram-negative organisms, which are usually found in the anal area, are most frequently implicated.

FAST FACTS in a NUTSHELL

Prevention of UTIs:

- Cleanse perineum with each diaper change
- Wipe perineum from front to back
- Avoid bubble baths
- Have child urinate immediately after a bath
- Wear white, cotton underwear
- Use loose-fitting pants

Description

- May involve the urethra, bladder, ureters, and kidney
- Uncircumcised male infants younger than 3 months are at highest risk
- May be present with or without symptoms
- Urinary stasis is the single most important factor influencing occurrence

Manifestations

- Neonatal symptoms: Poor feeding, dehydration, vomiting, rapid respirations, screaming on urination, jaundice, seizures, and enlarged bladder or kidneys
- Infancy symptoms (1 to 24 months): Poor feeding, vomiting, excessive thirst, straining or screaming with urination, foul-smelling urine, persistent diaper rash, pallor, fever, seizures, and enlarged bladder or kidneys
- Childhood symptoms (2 years or older): Poor appetite, vomiting, excessive thirst, enuresis, incontinence or frequent urination, painful urination, edema, pallor, fatigue, blood in urine, abdominal or back pain, hypertension, and seizures

An assessment for UTI should be done if the child exhibits any of the following symptoms:

- Incontinence (in toilet-trained child)
- Strong-smelling urine
- Frequency or urgency

Diagnostic Criteria

- History and presenting symptoms
- Urine culture (catheterized specimen recommended)
- Dipstick of urine for leukocyte esterase or nitrite (for quick assessment)

Interventions

- Eliminate current infection
  - Antimicrobial drugs: Penicillin, sulfonamide (trimethoprim and sulfisoxazole in combination), cephalosporins, and nitrofurantoin
- Frequent, complete emptying of the bladder to avoid over-distention and/or stasis

≡ *FAST FACTS in a NUTSHELL*

To approximate bladder capacity of a child use the following formula:

Age in years + 2 ounces = bladder volume

- Encourage fluids
- Keep urine acidic (pH of 6)
  - Suggest acid-ash producing foods: meats, cheese, prunes, apple juice, cranberry juice, plums, and whole grains
- Avoid constipation
- Prevent systemic spread of infection
  - Follow-up study (reculture) after treatment
- Preserve renal function
  - Recurrent infections can result in renal scarring

- Identify contributing factors to reduce recurrence
  - Anatomical defects such as primary reflux may need treatment

Defects

Congenital external defects of the genitourinary system can have a serious psychological impact on the child if not managed as early as possible. Following are some of the most common of these defects:

Hydrocele: Fluid in the scrotum. Manifests as an enlarged scrotum that lights up when a flashlight is focused behind the scrotal sac. Surgical repair would be indicated if spontaneous resolution does not occur in 1 year.

Hypospadias: Urethral opening is located behind the glans penis or anywhere along the ventral surface of the penile shaft. Circumcision is postponed until decision is made regarding need for surgical correction, which may include penile and urethral lengthening and bladder neck reconstruction.

- The objectives of surgical correction may include enabling child to stand to void and provide direct stream of urine, improve physical appearance of genitalia, and produce a sexually adequate organ.

Epispadias: Urethral opening located on dorsal surface of the penis (see hypospadias).

Cryptorchidism: Failure of one or both testes to descend through the inguinal canal as detected by manual palpation.

- Objectives for treatment include prevention of damage to the testicle, decrease the incidence of malignant tumor formation, avoid trauma or torsion, close the inguinal canal, and provide cosmetic repair.
  - Medical treatment—administration of human chorionic gonadotropin (HCG)
  - Surgical treatment—orchiopexy

GLOMERULAR DISEASE

Glomerular disease is a large group of diseases that are caused by systemic disease or infection, or that can be associated with hereditary disorders. Disorders in this category impact the glomerulus of the kidneys. The glomerular membrane, which is normally impermeable to proteins, becomes permeable to proteins such as albumin. Albumin is lost in the urine, causing hyperalbuminuria, which in turn lowers blood levels, resulting in hypoalbuminemia. Following are the most common of these diseases.

Nephrotic Syndrome/Nephrosis

Description

- Noninflammatory degenerative kidney disease distinguished by the presence of increased amounts of protein in the urine
- Can occur as:
  - Primary disease, idiopathic nephrosis, childhood nephrosis, or minimal-change nephrotic syndrome (MCNS)
  - Congenital form inherited as an autosomal recessive disorder
- More common between 2 and 7 years of age
- Twice as likely in males.
- If detected early, 80% of affected children will have a favorable prognosis

Manifestations

- Weight gain
- Edema; periorbital, facial, scrotal, feet, abdominal ascities; and pleural effusion
- Irritability, easily fatigued
- Anorexia
- Relapses can occur over many years

=======================*FAST FACTS in a NUTSHELL*

No vaccines or immunizations are given during the acute stage of nephrosis.

Diagnostic Criteria

- History and clinical symptoms
- Proteinuria
- Reduced serum albumin levels

Interventions

- The objective of therapeutic management includes:
  - Reduce excretion of urinary protein
  - Reduce fluid retention
  - Prevent infection
  - Minimize complications
- Corticosteroids (prednisone) usually 2 mg/kg body weight/day for 6 weeks followed by 1.5 mg/kg every other day for 6 weeks
- Monitor fluid retention and excretion through intake and output, and daily weight
- Prevent infection (frequent handwashing, avoid contact with illness)
- Manage diet, give preferred foods to increase appetite, restrict salt

Acute Glomerulonephritis/Acute Poststreptococcal Glomerulonephritis (Bright's Disease)

Description

- May be a primary event or associated as a postinfection syndrome
- Acute poststreptococcal glomerulonephritis is the most common postinfectious renal disease in childhood
- Allergic immune reaction after group A beta-hemolytic streptococcal infection
- Most common between 3 and 7 years of age with peak onset at 6 to 7 years of age

Manifestations

- Latent period of 10 to 21 days occurs between the streptococcal infection and the onset of clinical symptoms
- Oliguria
- Periorbital edema
- Hyperkalemia
- Hypertension and circulatory congestion
- Hematuria (smoky-brown or bloody urine) and proteinuria

Diagnostic Criteria

- Urinalysis reveals presence of red blood cells and protein (3+ or 4+)

- Circulating serum antibodies to streptococci
- Blood urea nitrogen, creatinine, erythrocyte sedimentation rate, and potassium levels are all elevated

═══════════════════════════*FAST FACTS in a NUTSHELL*

Since excessive potassium in the blood can produce cardiac toxicity, potatoes, bananas, and other high-potassium foods should be restricted until oliguria is resolved.

Interventions

- Antibiotic therapy if evidence of persistent streptococcal infection
- Relieve symptoms
  - Bed rest until hematuria resolves
  - Sodium- and potassium-restrictive diet until edema and oliguria resolved
  - Diuretics and antihypertensive drugs for the management of elevated blood pressure
- Recovery is usually spontaneous and complete

OTHER RENAL DISORDERS

Wilms' Tumor/Nephroblastoma

Description

- Most common malignant renal and intraabdominal tumor of childhood
- Peak age of diagnosis is 3 years of age, rarely seen after 5 years of age
- Familial origin arising in utero
- Left kidney favored but can affect both kidneys
- Prognosis and survival rates are highest (90%) with localized tumor stage I or II

Manifestations

- Abdominal mass or enlargement
- Weight loss

- Anemia
- Hypertension

FAST FACTS in a NUTSHELL

Do NOT palpate the abdomen if Wilm's tumor is suspected. Care is taken in the bathing and handling of the child to prevent trauma to the tumor site and/or disseminate cancer cells to adjacent tissues.

Diagnostic Criteria

- History and physical exam
- Abdominal ultrasound or computed tomography (CT) scan
- IV pyelogram

Interventions

- Surgery as soon as possible for removal of tumor, affected kidney, and adjacent adrenal gland
- Chemotherapy is indicated for all stages
- Radiotherapy is indicated for large tumors or metastasis

CONCLUSION

Although many diseases of the genitourinary system in children are present when a child is born, some disorders develop as the child grows. The nursing management of these disorders vastly differs from that for adults and presents a unique challenge to the pediatric nurse.

REFERENCES AND FURTHER READING

Hockenberry, M., & Wilson, D. (2013). *Wong's essentials of pediatric nursing* (9th ed.). St. Louis, MO: Elsevier.

Leifer, G. (2011). *Introduction to maternity & pediatric nursing* (6th ed.). St. Louis, MO: Elsevier.

Urology: Genitourinary and kidney disorders. (n.d.). Retrieved from http://www.chw.org/display/PPF/DocID/22605/router.asp

19

Musculoskeletal Disorders

Musculoskeletal disorders are some of the most common causes of illness and hospitalization in children due to their active nature. Pediatric clients with neurological impairment may also have impairment of the musculoskeletal system; however, pediatric clients with musculoskeletal impairments can see improvement made through the refinement of the nervous system. After studying this chapter, you will have a basic understanding of the most common musculoskeletal disorders found in children.

This chapter reviews:

1. Common pediatric musculoskeletal disorders
2. Etiology of pediatric musculoskeletal disorders
3. Pediatric-specific care of musculoskeletal disorders

VARIATIONS IN PEDIATRIC ANATOMY AND PHYSIOLOGY

The musculoskeletal system supports the body structure and provides for client movement. Skeletal growth is most rapid during infancy and adolescence. The primary difference between the pediatric and adult skeletal systems lies in the fact that pediatric bone is not ossified, epiphyses are present, and the periosteum is thicker and produces callus more rapidly. Injury to the epiphysis can affect bone growth. Other musculoskeletal differences include the following:

- Bones of children are more resilient, allowing the bone to bend before a break occurs
- Bones in children heal quickly due to the rich blood supply and osteogenic activity
- Musculoskeletal discomfort commonly called "growing pains" may be growth related
- With the rapid growth of the skeletal frame, deformities may become more severe

MUSCULOSKELETAL DISORDERS

The most common pediatric musculoskeletal disorders involve pediatric trauma. A pediatric client can experience soft tissue injuries with or without traumatic fractures. A fracture occurs when the resistance between a bone and an applied stress results in the disruption in the integrity of the bone. It is mainly caused by accidents.

Soft Tissue Injuries

Description

- Contusion: A tearing of the subcutaneous tissue, which results in hemorrhage, edema, and pain. A hematoma is a common finding from the leakage of blood into the soft tissue.
- Sprain: A torn or stretched ligament away from the bone at the point of trauma, causing damage to blood vessels, muscles, and nerves. Swelling, inability to put weight on limb, and pain are common.
- Strain: A microscopic tear to the muscle or tendon may occur over time, causing chronic symptoms of edema and pain.

Manifestations

- Edema
- Hematoma
- Inability to complete normal activities
- Pain

Diagnosis

- Radiographic studies
- Computed tomography (CT)
- Magnetic resonance imaging (MRI)

Interventions

- Apply cold/ice pack; alternate cold/ice pack in 30-minute intervals
- Elevate extremity above the heart
- Apply elastic bandage; perform neurovascular checks

══ *FAST FACTS in a NUTSHELL*

Instruct parents on the principle of soft tissue management with the following mnemonic:

Rest
Ice
Compression
Elevation

Traumatic Fractures

A fracture should be strongly suspected when an infant/toddler refuses to walk or crawl.

Description

- Greenstick: An incomplete fracture where one side of the bone is broken and the other side is bent. Pediatric clients have bones that are soft, flexible, and more likely to splinter
- Simple or closed: Bone is broken but the skin over the bone is not
- Compound or open: A wound in the skin is accompanied by a broken bone. Due to the open area, an additional risk of infection is present
- Spiral: Occurs from a twisting motion; common with physical abuse
- Complicated fracture: Fracture results in injury to other organs/tissues
- Buckle (torus): A bulge or raised area at fracture

Manifestations

- Deformity: Visible bone through skin, abnormal rotation of an extremity, shortened extremity
- Crepitus: Grating sound from two bones rubbing together
- Visible muscle spasms: Resulting from the pulling forces over the bone, misalignment
- Ecchymosis: Bleeding into the soft tissues
- Edema: Resulting from the trauma to the bone and tissues

Diagnosis

- Radiographic studies: Must remain still during procedure; sedate if necessary

Interventions

- Neurovascular checks
  - Pain: Use pediatric age-appropriate pain scale
  - Sensation: Check numbness and tingling or loss of sensation
  - Skin temperature: Should be warm to touch
  - Skin color: Observe distal to injury for changes
  - Capillary refill: Normal within 3 seconds
  - Pulses: Compare with unaffected extremity; palpable and strong
  - Movement: Should be able to move during passive motion
- Clean wound, if appropriate
- Monitor vital signs, pain, and neurological status; keep the client warm
- Stabilize the area; maintain alignment; place the client in the supine position
- Administer analgesics; use age-appropriate distractions

FAST FACTS in a NUTSHELL

Most fractures are casted.

- Plaster of Paris casts are heavy, not water resistant, with a prolonged drying time of up to 12 hours.
- Synthetic fiberglass casts are light, water resistant, and dry within 30 minutes.

Pain and a compromised neurovascular status should be immediately reported, as these may be signs of compartment syndrome. Recall the 6 Ps: Pain, Pulselessness, Pallor, Paresthesia, Paralysis, Pressure.

- Casting considerations: Position on a pillow; keep elevated and rotate until dry; handle cast with palm of hand until dry; complete neurovascular checks; keep casts dry
- Traction is used infrequently in pediatrics as newer technology has produced orthopedic fixation devices that allow partial or full mobility, preventing long-term immobilization. Also, surgical intervention may be carried out soon after the fracture

BIRTH AND DEVELOPMENTAL DEFECTS

Some defects are identified at birth or soon after. Skilled assessment is necessary to identify defects early so treatment can be started.

Developmental Dysplasia of the Hip (DDH)

A spectrum of disorders related to abnormal development of the hip.

Description

There are two major groups:

- Idiopathic: The client is neurologically intact
- Teratologic: Involves a neuromuscular defect

There are three degrees of developmental dysplasia of the hip:

- Acetabular dysplasia: Delay in acetabular development; mildest form
- Subluxation: Incomplete dislocation of the hip; a middle stage between dysplasia and complete dislocation; most common
- Dislocation: Femoral head loses contact with the acetabulum; most severe form

Manifestations in the Infant

- Asymmetry of the gluteal and thigh folders
- Positive Ortolani and Barlow tests
- Limited hip abduction
- Shortening of the femur

Manifestations in the Child

- Walks with a limp
- One leg shorter than the other
- Walking on the toes of one foot
- Pelvis shifts downward when weight is applied

Diagnosis

- Ortolani and Barlow click
- Ultrasound
- Radiographic study

Interventions

- Newborn to 6 months
  - Pavlik harness: Wear for 12 hours, adjust straps to maintain positioning, educate on skin care under harness
  - Bryant traction: A type of skin traction; hips flexed at 90-degree angle; perform neurovascular checks
  - Hip spica cast: Needs adjusted for growth; perform neurovascular checks; assess skin integrity and complete range of motion

Clubfoot

A complex deformity of the ankle and foot that includes forefoot adduction, midfoot supination, hindfootvarus, and ankle equinus. Most cases of clubfoot are a combination of these positions.

Description

Categorized as:

- Positional: From intrauterine crowding
- Syndromic: In association with other syndromes
- Congenital: Idiopathic

Manifestations

- The most common type of clubfoot is talipesequinovarus (TEV), in which the foot is pointed downward and inward

- Assessed at birth; feet can be manually moved toward a normal position due to the ability to bend bones but returns to prior deformity when released
- Can occur in one or both feet; categorized as positional

Diagnosis

- Upon position of ankles and feet; can be seen prenatally on ultrasound

Interventions

- Encourage bonding; have parents hold and cuddle
- Series of casting shortly after birth
  - Teach cast care; neurovascular checks; skin integrity
- Surgical interventions of congenital/syndromic clubfoot
  - Osteotomy: Removing bone
  - Fusion: Adhering two or more bones together
  - Tendon lengthening or shortening
  - Monitor growth and development

Torticolis

Description

Torticollis (wry neck) is a symptom that causes a child's chin to be rotated to one side and the head to the other side. The child may cry if the head moves. The two most common disorders that can cause torticollis include:

- Congenital muscular torticollis: Symptoms are present at birth in which the sternocleidomastoid muscle is injured during the birth process or from the malformation of the spine. It can be associated with a breech for forceps delivery and may be seen in conjunction with other birth defects.
- Acquired torticollis: Seen in older children. It may be associated with cervical spine injury, inflammation, or neurological disorders.

Manifestations

- The infant holds the head to the opposite side involved; chin is tilted in the opposite direction

- Pain upon movement with acquired torticollis but no pain in the infant with congenital torticollis unless head moved in the opposite direction
- A hard, palpable mass of dense fibrotic tissue may be felt on assessment

Diagnosis

- Physical assessment findings
- Behavior of infant or child
- Cervical spine radiographs or a CT scan

Interventions

- Passive stretching and range-of-motion exercises; physical therapy may be indicated; surgical release of the sternocleidomastoid may be required
- Playing a game or sitting on the affected side to encourage the infant to turn in that direction; can lead to positional plagiocephaly and facial asymmetry if the child lays in the same position
- Refer any infant and child with symptoms to a physician for further follow-up
- Instruct on Tylenol or pain relievers to ensure an accurate dose; supervise using a heating pad

Scoliosis

Scoliosis is a lateral curvature of the spine that exceeds 10 degrees and can also cause rib asymmetry.
  Scoliosis can be:

- Congenital: Early diagnosis
- Associated: Associated with other disorders
- Idiopathic: Caused during adolescence; most common form; may be genetic

Description

- Asymmetry in the scapula, ribs, flanks, shoulders, and hips

Manifestations

- Improperly fitting clothing
- One leg shorter than the other

Diagnosis

- Radiographs
- Assessment: Screen preadolescents by having the child bend at the waist with arms hanging down and observe for asymmetry; measure truncal rotation with a scoliometer; assess for respiratory impairment

Interventions

- Depends on the degree, location, and type of curvature
- Bracing: Slows the progression of curve
  - Assist with fitting of the brace; assess skin integrity; teach application of brace
- Surgical intervention: Used for curvature greater than 45 degrees
  - Spinal fusion with rod placement; monitor pain, may need ICU postoperatively, turn using log rolling method, emphasize physical therapy

DISORDERS AND DYSFUNCTION OF THE MUSCULOSKELETAL SYSTEM

While bone is typically thought of as lifeless and unchanging, bone is actually living tissue with a function within our body system.

Osteomyelitis

Osteomyelitis is an infection of the bone that occurs most often in infancy or between the ages of 5 and 14 years. Osteomyelitis can stem from an injury to the bone itself, an open fracture contaminating the bone, surgery, or infection spreading from a distant site.

Description

- Long bones contain few phagocytic cells
- *Staphylococcus aureus* is the organism responsible in most children over 5 years; *Haemophilus influenzae* is the most common cause in infants and young children
- Inflammation causes exudates that collect under the bone marrow in the cortex of the bone creating an abscess
- IV drug users often develop *Salmonella* and *Pseudomonas*

Manifestations

- Pain and ischemia from compression of vessels in the area
- An elevated periosteum due to pus formation; possible septic arthritis in the joint due to the spread of infection
- Decrease in voluntary movement of the extremity; a limp with lower extremity compromise; muscle spasms; limited range of motion

Diagnosis

- Blood cultures to identify the primary infection
- Urine culture; blood chemistry; microbiology culture of fluid
- Radiographic study

Interventions

- Prompt and aggressive treatment is needed to decrease complications; joint aspiration may be needed to drain pus and prevent bone necrosis
- Monitor vital signs
- Intravenous antibiotics possibly lasting 4 to 6 weeks
- Pain management and range of motion; ensure appropriate dosage
- Bed rest or wheelchair use until able to bear weight

Muscular Dystrophy

A group of disorders that include progressive muscle degeneration in primarily the skeletal (voluntary) muscles. The childhood form, Duchenne's muscular dystrophy, is the most common.

Description

- Incidence in 1:3,600 live male births; occurs in all races/ethnic groups; sex-linked (males only); inherited
- Dystrophin, a protein in skeletal muscle, is absent; critical for maintenance for muscle cells; skeletal muscle fibers are affected but not the spinal cord or peripheral nerves
- There is no cure and is typically fatal by 20 to 25 years of age

Manifestations

- Onset between 2 and 6 years; however, delayed motor development may be seen during infancy; hips, thighs, pelvis, and shoulders are affected initially
- Progressive weakness; clumsiness; falling; contractures of the ankles and hips; Gowers' maneuver is noted, which is a characteristic way of rising from the floor
- The disease becomes progressively worse, leading to wheelchair dependence; death typically occurs from cardiac failure or respiratory tract infection

Diagnosis

- A serum blood polymerase chain reaction (PCR) is diagnostic
- Marked increase in serum creatine phosphokinase
- Muscle biopsy reveals degeneration of the muscle fibers with replacement by fat and connective tissue; DNA testing reveals the presence of the gene
- A myelogram showing decreases in the amplitude and duration of motor unit ability

Interventions

- Treatment is supportive to prevent contractures and maintain quality of life; promote mobility
- Corticosteroids may slow progression; calcium supplements are prescribed to prevent osteoporosis; antidepressants for the chronic and debilitating state of the disease
- Braces, orthopedic aids, and positioning aids become necessary
- Contractions and spinal curvatures may need surgical interventions
- Encourage passive stretching or strengthening exercises; alternate periods of rest with periods of activity
- Assess cardiac and lung fields; position for maximum lung expansion, usually upright
- Offer support to client and family; refer to the Muscular Dystrophy Association

Juvenile Idiopathic Arthritis

Description

- An autoimmune disorder in which the client's antibodies mainly target the joints
- Chronic disease with healthy periods alternating with flare-ups in symptoms
- For some, the disease resolves by adolescence or adulthood; others have symptoms throughout adulthood
- Other nonjoint manifestations include: malaise, poor appetite, poor weight gain/growth, systemic changes
- Types include:
  - Pauciarticular: Most common; less than four joints involved; complications include uneven leg bone growth
  - Polyarticular: Involvement of five or more joints; may involve small joints; complications include a progressive form of arthritis; joint damage and rheumatoid nodules may occur
  - Systemic: In addition to joint damage, fever and rash may be present; liver, spleen, and lymph node involvement my occur; complications extend to the heart and lungs

Manifestations

- Inflammation in the joint causes pain, erythema, warmth, stiffness, and swelling
- Client experiences stiffness in the morning due to inactivity at night; difficult to get out of bed and ready for school

Diagnosis

- Assessment of physical symptoms
- Serum chemistry; complete blood count identifying anemia; elevated erythrocyte sedimentation rate; positive antinuclear antibody in young children with pauciarticular form or positive rheumatoid factor in adolescents with polyarticular disease

Interventions

- Encourage regular pediatric rheumatologist and ophthalmologist visits

- Maintain joint range of motion and muscle strength; use splints to prevent contractures; physical therapy and occupational therapy may be helpful
- Encourage warm baths, massage, and comfort measures to relieve pain and promote rest
- Instruct teachers, coaches, classmates, and mentors about limitations of disease

Legg-Calve-Perthes Disease

Description

- Blood supply is interrupted to the epiphysis; tissue death occurs called avascular necrosis; in turn, it affects the development of the head of the femur

Manifestations

- A painless limp and restricted range of motion
- Healing occurs spontaneously over 2 to 4 years but there may remain a marked distortion of the head of the femur, causing an imperfect joint; degenerative arthritis may occur in adulthood
- Discomfort occurs in boys between the ages of 5 and 12 years
- Typically unilateral

Diagnosis

- Radiograph evaluation
- Bone scan

Interventions

- Self-limiting disorder; treatment involves keeping the femoral head deep in the hip socket during healing
- No weight bearing during healing; abduction casts or braces prevent subluxation, enabling the acetabulum to mold the head, preventing deformity

When partial immobility occurs, encourage:

- High-fiber diet
- Small, frequent meals
- Increase fluids
- Regular skin assessment
- Alternate school activities
- Age-appropriate diversional activity

Slipped Femoral Capital Epiphysis

Description

- Spontaneous displacement of the epiphysis of the femur; most often occurs during periods of rapid growth such as in the preadolescent
- The epiphysis of the femur widens, femoral head and epiphysis remain in the acetabulum; head of femur rotates and then displaces
- Not related to trauma

Manifestations

- Thigh pain, limp, inability to bear weight on the affected leg

Diagnosis

- Radiograph evaluation confirms

Interventions

- Traction to maintain placement then surgery for screw insertion
- Assess for complications of impaired circulation to the epiphysis, which can lead to necrosis of the head of the femur

REFERENCES AND FURTHER READING

Hockenberry, M., & Wilson, D. (2013). *Wong's essentials of pediatric nursing* (9th ed.). St. Louis, MO: Elsevier.

Leifer, G. (2011). *Introduction to maternity & pediatric nursing* (6th ed.). St. Louis, MO: Elsevier.

20

Metabolic Disorders

The endocrine or ductless glands work with the nervous system to regulate the body's metabolic processes. Hormones are the chemical substances produced by the glands. Hormones interact with specific target organs to create an effect on the body. Too much or too little of a given hormone may result in a disease state. After reviewing this chapter, you will have a basic understanding of the most common metabolic disorders found in children.

This chapter reviews:

1. Pathophysiology behind the metabolic system in pediatric clients
2. Nursing care required for pediatric clients with various metabolic conditions
3. Instruction necessary for families of clients with metabolic conditions

VARIATIONS IN PEDIATRIC ANATOMY AND PHYSIOLOGY

Most of the glands and structures of the endocrine system develop during the first trimester of fetal development. Hormonal control is immature until approximately 18 months of age, leaving the infant prone to dysfunction of the endocrine system. Since the newborn is supplemented by maternal hormones that cross the placental barrier, assessment begins with determining maternal endocrine functioning.

- Early signs of inborn metabolic errors include lethargy, poor feeding, failure to thrive, vomiting, and an enlarged liver
- An infection or body stress can precipitate symptoms of a latent defect in the older child
- Unexplained intellectual disability, a variety of developmental delay symptoms, seizures, nausea/vomiting, and an unexplained odor to the urine or body are considered subtle signs

Inborn Errors of Metabolism

Hundreds of hereditary biochemical disorders affect the metabolism. The disorders are autosomal recessive and can range in severity. As the infant adjusts to life, symptoms can rapidly emerge that are life-threatening.

Tay-Sachs Disease

Description

- Deficiency of hexosaminidase, an enzyme necessary for the metabolism of fats, causing lipid deposits to accumulate on nerve cells

Manifestations

- Infant appears normal until 5 to 6 months, when physical development slows (head lag, inability to sit)
- Mental decline and physical deterioration occur
- Blindness due to deposits on the optic nerve

Diagnosis

- Autosomal recessive trait in the Ashkenazi Jewish population
- Occurrence in 1:4,000 live births

Interventions

- Palliative care for the client; there is no treatment available
- Support for family; genetic and prenatal testing are available

Galactosemia

The body is unable to use the carbohydrates galactose and lactose. Symptoms begin when the newborn begins breastfeeding or ingesting formula.

Description

- Due to an error in enzyme function, there is an increase in the amount of galactose in the blood and urine resulting in cirrhosis of the liver, cataracts, and intellectual disability, if left untreated

Manifestations

- Early signs consist of lethargy, vomiting, hypotonia, diarrhea, and failure to thrive; signs begin abruptly and worsen gradually
- Jaundice occurs from liver disease

Diagnosis

- By observing galactosemia, galactosuria, and evidence of decreased enzyme activity in the red blood cells
- Screening tests are available

Interventions

- Instruct on eliminating milk- and lactose-containing products from the diet
- The nursing mother must discontinue breastfeeding; lactose-free and soy products are substituted
- Support parents as they learn to manage the disease process

Phenylketonuria (PKU)

A genetic disorder caused by faulty metabolism of phenylalanine, an amino acid that is essential to life and found in all protein foods.

Description

- Classic PKU is associated with blood phenylalanine levels over 20 mg/dL and can result in intellectual disability
- Less severe forms are now designated as "atypical PKU" or "mild hyperphenylalaninemia"
- The infant appears normal at birth but delayed development noted at 4 to 6 months

Manifestations

- When the infant is fed formula, phenylalanine accumulates in the blood
- Phenylpyruvic acid is found in the urine within the first weeks of life
- Failure to thrive, eczema, and skin conditions may exists; seizures occur in one third of the children

Diagnosis

- Guthrie blood test: Blood is obtained from a heel stick and placed on filter paper; obtained at 48 to 72 hours of life, preferably after ingestion of proteins
- Early diagnosis is paramount; by the time the urine test is positive, brain damage has occurred
- Mainly found in blonde and blue-eyed infants

Interventions

- Monitor blood levels of phenylalanine
- Teach dietary management; foods with low phenylalanine level with enough protein for growth and development of tissue; best to keep serum phenylalanine levels between 2 mg/dL and 10 mg/dL
- Breast milk has low phenylalanine levels; formulas such as Lofenalac and Phenex-1 have low levels
- Phenyl-free diet is introduced between ages 3 and 8 years; consult a dietician for menu options

FAST FACTS in a NUTSHELL

NutraSweet (aspartame) must be avoided as it is converted to phenylalanine.

Maple Syrup Urine Disease

Caused by a defect in the metabolism of branched-chain amino acids.

Description

- Causes marked serum elevations of leucine, isoleucine, and valine resulting in acidosis, cerebral degeneration, and death within 2 weeks of life if untreated

Manifestations

- Appears healthy at birth but soon develops feeding difficulties, loss of Moro reflex, hypotonia, irregular respirations, and convulsions
- The infant's urine, sweat, and cerumen have a characteristic maple syrup odor—a fruity odor due to ketoacidosis

Diagnosis

- Confirmed by blood and urine tests

Interventions

- Early detection is extremely important; report a urine with a sweet aroma
- Hydration and peritoneal dialysis reduces the amino acids and their metabolites from the blood
- Instruct on life-long low amounts of the amino acids leucine, isoleucine, and valine; leucin levels frequently cause exacerbations
- Instruct client on how to prevent infections, which can cause an exacerbation of the disease

Endocrine Disorders

Endocrine disorders affect how the body runs and how the client feels. Disorders may have an insidious onset. Several disorders are highlighted; however, the most common endocrine disorder is diabetes.

Hyperthyroidism

Hyperthyroidism occurs when the thyroid gland makes too much thyroxin. Hyperthyroidism is less common in children and adolescents than it is in adults. Neonates are tested to determine thyroid levels after birth.

Description

- Hyperthyroidism leads to an increased metabolism and affects many cells and tissues throughout the body, including the brain, heart, bone, skin, and intestinal tract

Manifestations

- Bulging eyes (exophthalmos); rapid pulse; heat intolerance
- Nervousness and difficulty concentrating; increased perspiration; difficulty sleeping
- In infants younger than 3 years, high thyroid hormone levels can result in cognitive delay
- Development of a goiter

Diagnosis

- In older children, the most common cause of hyperthyroidism is Graves's disease, an autoimmune disorder
- In newborns, the most common cause of an overactive thyroid is neonatal Graves's disease, which is a temporary condition
- Assessment of the thyroid gland
- Serum thyroid studies; thyroid scan

Interventions

- Intervention depends on treatment plan of:
  - Oral medication therapy
  - Radiation therapy
  - Surgical removal of thyroid
- Monitor antithyroid drug therapy and serum laboratory studies
- Instruct on radioactive iodine therapy if needed
- Wound care for thyroidectomy incision

Hypothyroidism

Occurs when there is a deficiency in the secretions of the thyroid gland (T3 and T4). A common pediatric disorder of the endocrine system. Classified as two types:

- Congenital hypothyroidism: The gland is absent at birth or not functioning; lifelong treatment is required
- Acquired hypothyroidism or juvenile hypothyroidism: Acquired by the older child; intellectual disability and neurological complications are not seen in the older child

Description

- Most often occurs during period of rapid growth
- Symptoms similar to adults such as feeling tired, weak, or not able to tolerate the cold

Manifestations

- Intellectual disability, if untreated
- Short stature, growth failure, delayed physical maturation and development
- Reduced activity; sluggishness; sleeps a lot; weight gain
- Enlarged tongue; poor eating; difficulty breathing, including during sleep
- Dry skin; hands and feet are cold
- Hypotonia of musculoskeletal system and intestinal tract; constipation

Diagnosis

- Early diagnosis is important to prevent developing complications
- Serum thyroid levels; thyroid ultrasound or scan

Interventions

- Instruction of daily medication therapy of synthetic hormone sodium levothyroxine
- Monitor frequent thyroid function tests
- Medication therapy reverses symptoms and prevents further mental retardation
- Instruct to administer medication at same time each day

- Instruct on signs of toxicity such as restlessness, weight loss, irritability, and hair loss
- Monitor growth charts; encourage medical identification bracelet

FAST FACTS in a NUTSHELL

Thyroid medication absorption is affected by soy-based formulas and fiber and iron preparations. Therefore, carefully assess for infant formulas such as Similac Soy, Isomil, and Prosobee (American Academy of Pediatrics, 2008)

Diabetes Insipidus

Diabetes insipidus is the consequence of posterior pituitary hypofunction, which results in a decreased secretion of vasopressin, the antidiuretic hormone (ADH). A lack of ADH results in uncontrolled diuresis, as the kidney does not concentrate the urine during dehydration episodes.

Description

Classified into two types:
- Central: Disorder of the posterior pituitary; most common form.
- Nephrogenic: Not associated with the pituitary gland but related to a decrease in the sensitivity to antidiuretic hormone. Transmitted genetically or acquired by chronic renal disease, hypercalcemia, hypokalemia, or possible drug interactions.

Manifestations

- Abrupt onset of excessive thirst; drinking an increased amount of water
- Excessive urination not related to a decrease in fluid intake; enuresis
- Weight loss; failure to thrive in infants; decreased fontanels
- Commonly occurs following complications from head trauma or cranial surgery to remove hypothalamic pituitary tumors; 10% of cases in children are idiopathic

Diagnosis

- Radiographic studies of the skull and kidney to determine the presence of a tumor
- Serum blood levels of a deficiency of ADH; elevated sodium level
- Fluid deprivation test measuring vasopressin release

Interventions

- In neonates and infants, treatment is fluid therapy; in older children, treatment is hormone replacement of vasopressin
- Assessment: vital signs, intake and output (hourly)
- Note any signs of dehydration (increased respiratory rate, tachycardia, skin turgor)
- Early signs of dehydration may include fever, irritability, vomiting, and constipation
- Monitor lab results:
  - Urinalysis: urine is dilute; specific gravity is less than 1.005
  - Chemistry, including sodium and potassium
- Promote hydration: maintain fluid regimen, discourage diuretic drinks
- Feed infants more frequently; may need to be awakened for fluid at night
- Teach regarding desmopressin acetate (which is the trademark DDAVP, intranasal. parenteral, or oral administration); it is a long acting vasopressin analogue. The dose depends on the child's age (typically for children over 3 years of age), urine output, and urine-specific gravity

=== *FAST FACTS in a NUTSHELL*

Question: What are the considerations for lifelong DDAVP use?

Answer: The nurse must provide specific directions for medication use:

- Monitor blood pressure; instruct on norms
- Note signs of overdose, which are similar to those of water intoxication; that is, edema, lethargy, nausea, depressed central nervous system
- Purchase a medical identification bracelet; notify those with frequent contact
- Discuss condition with school nurse for considerations of frequent bathroom use and increase water ingestion

Diabetes Mellitus (DM)

A common, chronic disease of childhood where carbohydrate, protein, and lipid metabolism are impaired. If symptoms go unrecognized, diabetic ketoacidosis (DKA) develops, resulting in anorexia, nausea, or vomiting; ketones in the urine; and sweet-smelling breath. When the condition becomes life-threatening, symptoms progress to Kussmaul respirations or air hunger, progressing to coma and death. Pediatric considerations include:

- Clients perform blood glucose monitoring more often due to activity
- Clients need to keep an activity, diet, and blood glucose diary
- Clients use a sliding scale to calculate insulin dosage or an insulin pump
- Clients need sufficient calories and good nutrition; education needed
- Adjustments need to be made in insulin during holidays, school parties/trips
- Responsible adults need to be aware of diabetic status when parents are not present
- Before athletic practices, add an extra snack containing 15 to 30 g carbohydrate for each hour of exercise; have readily accessible glucose tablets

Description

The major forms of diabetes are termed:

- Type 1: Caused by a deficiency of insulin secretion due to pancreatic beta cell damage; an autoimmune disorder
- Type 2: A consequence of insulin resistance that occurs at the level of skeletal muscle, liver, and adipose tissue with different degrees of beta cell impairment. Historically type 2 has occurred in adults, but the incidence has been increasing in children
- Other causes of insulin deficiency include: diseases of the exocrine gland, drug or chemical interactions, genetic defects/syndromes, infection, or gestational diabetes

Hypoglycemia: Blood glucose levels under 70 mg/dL with symptoms including:	Hyperglycemia: Blood glucose levels over 200 mg/dL with symptoms including:
Diaphoresis	Dry, flushed skin
Tremors, shakiness	Blurred vision
Palpations, tachycardia	Abdominal cramping, nausea/vomiting, fruity breath
Confusion, disorientation	Mental changes, irritability, fatigue/weakness
Slurred speech	Polydipsia, polyuria, polyphagia

Diagnosis

- Blood glucose levels to monitor glycemic control; urine ketone testing
- Hemoglobin A1c levels
  - Infants to 6 years of age: HbA1c less than 8.5%
  - 6 to 12 years: HbA1c less than 8%
  - 13 to 19 years: HbA1c less than 7.5%
- Assessment of client symptoms

Interventions

- Multidisciplinary health team and others including the client and family, school nurse, coaches, teachers; educate client and family for self-management
- Role play diabetic scenarios to see the family and client's reaction and problem-solving ability; promote confidence in ability to handle disease process; encourage support groups and camps
- Instruct on blood glucose monitoring, insulin administration, symptoms of hypoglycemia/hyperglycemia, calorie-controlled diet, exercise regimen
- Typically two to four injections are needed depending on the needs of the client; doses vary during times of infections, stress, or puberty; pediatric clients are prescribed the same types of insulin as adults (Table 20.1)
- Double check dosage with physician order and second nurse; rotate injection sites to avoid adipose hypertrophy, which causes fatty lumps and poor absorption

TABLE 20.1 Insulin

Insulin type	Name	Onset	Peak	Duration
Rapid acting	Aspart (NovoLog) Lispro (Humalog) Glulisine (Apidra)	Within 15 minutes	30–90 minutes	3–5 hours
Short acting	Regular (Humulin R) (Novolin R)	30–60 minutes	2–4 hours	5–8 hours
Intermediate acting	NPH (Humulin N) (Novolin N)	1–3 hours	2–4 hours	10–16 hours
Long acting (Not mixed with other insulin)	Glargine (Lantus) Detemir (Levemir)	1–2 hours	No peak; steady coverage	6–24 hours

- Monitor for complications such as electrolyte disturbances, acidosis, coma, hypo-/hyperglycemia
- Insulin pumps are also common in the pediatric population; pumps are used as a more physiological way to deliver insulin in the hope of improved long-term outcomes

FAST FACTS in a NUTSHELL

Blood glucose levels vary according to age. According to the American Diabetes Association (2011), normal levels for nondiabetics is 70 to 110 mg/dL.

- Under 6 years with type 1 DM: 100 to 180 mg/dL before meals; bedtime 110 to 200 mg/dL
- 6 to 12 years with type 1 DM: 90 to 180 mg.dL before meals; bedtime 100 to 180 mg/dL
- 13 to 19 years with type 1 DM: 90 to 130 mg/dL before meals; bedtime 90 to 150 mg/dL

American Diabetes Association. (2014). Retrieved from http://www.diabetes.org

Bhatia, J., & Greer, F. (2008). Use of soy protein-based formulas in infant feeding. *American Academy of Pediatrics, 121*(5), 1062–1068.

Hockenberry, M., & Wilson, D. (2013). *Wong's essentials of pediatric nursing* (9th ed.). St. Louis, MO: Elsevier.

Kaufman, F., Halvorson, M., Carpenter, S., Devoe, D., & Pitukcheewanont, P. (2001). Pump therapy for children: Weighing the risks and benefits. *Diabetes Spectrum, 14*(2), 84–89.

Leifer, G. (2011). *Introduction to maternity & pediatric nursing* (6th ed.). St. Louis, MO: Elsevier.

21

Sensory Disorders

There are significant differences between the child and adult in regard to eye and ear structures. The eustachian tube in infants is shorter, wider, and straighter than in older children and adults, and this structural difference contributes to infections in the ear. The walls of the ear canal are more pliable in newborns and young infants due to underdeveloped cartilage and bony structures, and the infant is unable to communicate the presence of painful disorders of the middle ear. In infants, the immature eye muscles allow the eyes to cross until about 6 weeks of age, and tears are scant or absent during the first month or so after birth (this is a normal phenomenon that should be shared with parents to decrease concern or anxiety). It is important for the pediatric nurse to understand normal functioning of the sensory system and to avoid later development of vision, hearing, and/or balance problems.

This chapter reviews:

1. Common childhood disorders of the ear
2. Common vision disorders
3. Common eye disorders associated with trauma, infection, or tumor

DISORDERS AND DYSFUNCTION OF THE EAR

Inflammation of the external and/or middle ear can result in an acute infection that can spread to other structures of the ear, nose, sinuses, or throat. These inflammatory processes are often painful for the child. A variety of organisms can be responsible for infections of the external and middle ear.

Otitis Externa—Swimmer's Ear

Description

- An acute infection of the external ear canal
- Often caused by prolonged exposure to moisture

Manifestations

- Pain and tenderness on manipulation of the pinna or tragus of the ear
- Erythema of the ear canal
- Itching in ear canal

Diagnosis

- History and presenting symptoms
- Normal appearance of tympanic membrane
- Rule out presence of foreign body or other causes

Interventions

- Relief of pain, edema, and itching (with acetaminophen, ibuprofen, or ear drops of Auralgan, corticosteroid otic drops)
- Irrigation of the external ear canal to remove debris
- Topical antibiotic otic drops (such as polymyxin, neomycin, ofloxacin, or ciprofloxacin)

To decrease the incidence of swimmer's ear, limit exposure to water and dry the external ear canal thoroughly. Irrigating the ear canal with a mixture of 1 part white vinegar and 1 part rubbing alcohol helps to promote drying and prevent growth of bacteria and fungi that cause swimmer's ear.

Acute Otitis Media (OM)

Description

- Inflammation of the middle ear cavity
- Infectious type is commonly caused by *Streptococcus pneumoniae* and *Haemophilus influenzae*
- Noninfectious type has unknown cause: may be due to blocked eustachian tubes from edema or upper respiratory infections (URIs), allergic rhinitis, enlarged adenoids, or from pooling of fluids in the pharyngeal cavity
- Most often occurs after URI and usually affects children between 6 and 24 months of age and in early childhood. Rarely seen after age 7 years
- Chronic or unresolved otitis media can result in the development of otitis media with effusion (OME), where fluid persists in the middle ear for weeks/months
- Can lead to hearing loss and speech impairment

Manifestations

- Purulent fluid accumulates in the small space of the middle ear chamber, causing pressure and pain
- Infants become irritable, pull at ears, roll head from side to side
- Temperature can go up to 104° F
- Postauricular and cervical lymph gland enlargement
- Rhinorrhea, vomiting and diarrhea, and other signs of URIs
- Loss of appetite, difficulty sucking/chewing
- Red, bulging tympanic membrane
- Hearing loss
- Perforation of the tympanic membrane may result

Diagnosis

- History and presenting symptoms
- Throat culture to determine causative agent

FAST FACTS in a NUTSHELL

Prevention of otitis media includes:

- Avoid exposure to second-hand smoke
- Avoid exposure to air pollution
- Keep the child up to date with recommended immunizations
- Bottle feed babies in the upright position

Interventions

- Broad-spectrum antibiotics (such as amoxicillin, Augmentin)
- Analgesics (such as acetaminophen, ibuprofen, or ear drops of Auralgan)
- Myringotomy with tympanostomy tubes for OME

DISORDERS AND DYSFUNCTION OF THE EYE

The eye is an organ of vision. By 2 to 4 months of age, an infant can follow moving objects and develop eye–hand coordination. Depth perception does not develop until 9 months of age. Disorders of the eye can result in impairment of vision.

Amblyopia—Lazy Eye

Description

- A reduction in or loss of vision that usually occurs in children who strongly favor one eye
- Usually develops before age of 6 years

Manifestations

- Noticeably favoring one eye or a tendency to bump into objects on one side
- Symptoms are not always obvious

Diagnosis

- Based on history and presenting symptoms
- When vision in the "normal eye" is at least two Snellen lines better than the affected eye

Interventions

- Early detection with goal of achieving equal vision in each eye
- Eye glasses for refractive errors or patching of "good eye"

Strabismus/Cross-Eye/Squint

Description

- A condition in which both eyes do not direct toward the same object
- Two types:
  - Nonparalytic: Constant deviation in the gaze
    - Caused by faulty insertion of eye muscle with normal extraocular muscles
  - Paralytic: Deviation in gaze with movement
    - Caused by weakness or paralysis of extraocular muscle
- The brain will disable one eye to provide a clear image
- Can result in amblyopia

Manifestations

- Tilting of the head or squinting to focus on an object
- Covering one eye to see
- Missing objects during reaching

Diagnosis

- Based on history and presenting symptoms
- Physical examination of the eye

Interventions

- Nonparalytic strabismus is treated with corrective eyeglasses
- Paralytic strabismus is treated with patching the unaffected eye
- Surgery is performed between 3 and 4 years of age if no improvement to prevent blindness in the affected eye

Chalazion

Description

- A cyst or small lump in the eyelid caused by obstruction of an oil-producing or meibomian gland

Manifestations

- Lump on the upper or lower eyelids
- Redness, swelling, and soreness

Diagnosis

- Physical examination of the eyelid with presence of a cyst

Interventions

- Warm compresses to the eyelid for 10 to 15 minutes four times daily
- Daily washing of the eye lashes with nontearing shampoo to prevent recurrence
- Surgical incision and drainage if lump persists

Conjunctivitis—Pinkeye

Description

- An inflammation of the conjunctiva
  - Caused by irritants or chlamydia in newborns, or bacterial or viral infections in older children
- Infectious forms of conjunctivitis are considered contagious for 24 hours or until antimicrobial therapy

Manifestations

- Itching, burning of the eye
- Redness, edema, and discharge
- Photophobia

Diagnosis

- Based on history and presenting symptoms
- Physical examination of the eye

Interventions

- Topical antibiotic eye drops (such as erythromycin ointment 0.5%, gentamycin 0.3% ointment/solution, or Neosporin ointment) as ordered for infections
- Relieve symptoms:
  - Irrigation for removing chemical irritants
  - Prevent rubbing
  - Warm compresses to the eye

Hyphema

Description

- A hemorrhage or presence of blood in the anterior chamber of the eye
- Usually results from a blunt or perforating ocular injury or forceful coughing

Manifestations

- Bright red or dark red spot in front of the lower portion of the iris

Diagnosis

- Inspection and examination of the eye
- Intraocular pressure measurement (tonometry)

Interventions

- Bed rest
- Decrease intraocular pressure by positioning (30- to 45-degree head of bed elevation)
- Evaluation by ophthalmologist (complication may result in vision loss)

Retinoblastoma

Description

- A malignant tumor of the retina of the eye
- There are hereditary and spontaneous forms
- Average age at diagnosis: 12 months for bilateral tumors, 21 months for unilateral tumors

Manifestations

- A yellowish-white reflex is seen in the pupil (cat's eye reflex)
- Loss of vision
- Strabismus, hyphema, or pain if tumor is advanced

Diagnosis

- Ophthalmologic evaluation
- MRI or ultrasound for tumor detection in the eye
- Presence of *RB1* gene in blood and/or tumor sample

Interventions

- Small tumors may be treated via laser photocoagulation to destroy the blood vessels supplying the tumor

FAST FACTS in a NUTSHELL

Clinical trials are testing new chemotherapy drugs that have better penetration into the eye, in an attempt to avoid radiation therapy or having to surgically remove the eyes.

- Larger tumors are treated with chemotherapy or external beam irradiation
- Enucleation of the eye, if no possibility of saving the vision or preventing metastasis

CONCLUSION

Many of the disorders of the ears and eyes in children occur during early childhood, when the child is unable to communicate the symptoms being experienced. It is essential that the nurse be able to recognize the need for further evaluation and/or treatment.

REFERENCES AND FURTHER READING

Hockenberry, M., & Wilson, D. (2013). *Wong's essentials of pediatric nursing* (9th ed.). St. Louis, MO: Elsevier.

Leifer, G. (2011). *Introduction to maternity & pediatric nursing* (6th ed.). St. Louis, MO: Elsevier.

National Cancer Institute at the National Institutes of Health. (2013). *Retinoblastoma treatment*. Retrieved from http://www.cancer.gov/cancertopics/types/retinoblastoma

22

Common Communicable Diseases of Childhood

Since the development and activation of immunological agents or vaccines, the incidence of communicable diseases in children has decreased over the years. However, given the sometimes rapid transmission of communicable diseases and the limited availability of vaccines in certain countries, the nurse must be familiar with the recognition and appropriate intervention for communicable diseases in children.

This chapter reviews:

1. Common communicable diseases found in children in the United States
2. Sexually transmitted infections (STIs)
3. Human immunodeficiency virus (HIV)

FAST FACTS in a NUTSHELL

The earliest age for a vaccine to be administered to a child is determined by the youngest age at which the child can respond by developing antibodies to that illness.

Chickenpox/Varicella

This is a common illness that causes an itchy rash and red spots or blisters (pox) all over the body.

Etiology

- Varicella zoster virus

Transmission

- Direct contact, droplet, and contaminated objects

Incubation

- 2 to 3 weeks (average 13 to 17 days)

Period of Communicability

- One day prior to eruption of lesions until all lesions have crusted

Manifestations

- Mild fever
- Rash on body: Macules, papules, vesicles, and scabs

FAST FACTS in a NUTSHELL

Macule: Flat, circular, reddened area on the skin
Papule: Elevated, circular, reddened area on the skin
Vesicle: Elevated, circular, reddened area on the skin that contains fluid
Pustule: Elevated, circular, reddened area on the skin that contains pus

Interventions

- Antiviral agent acyclovir
- Antihistamines or calamine lotion to relieve itching
- Trim fingernails to prevent scratching
- Do not remove scabs (may cause scarring)
- Isolate from others

Diphtheria

Although rare in the United States, where children are immunized, it is still common in developing countries. Diphtheria is an acute bacterial disease that can infect the body in two areas: respiratory and skin.

Etiology

• Corynebacterium diphtheria

Transmission

• Direct contact

Incubation

• 2 to 5 days

Period of Communicability

• 2 to 4 weeks (until three cultures are negative)

Manifestations

• Symptoms resemble the common cold, serosanguineous mucopurulent nasal discharge
• Sore throat, white or gray membrane in throat, low-grade fever, lymphadenitis
• Hoarseness, dyspneic retractions, cyanosis, potential airway obstruction

Interventions

• Antibiotics, maintain airway, humidified oxygen, bed rest

Fifth Disease/Erythema Infectiosum

This is a viral illness that produces a distinctive red rash on the face, body, arms, and legs.

Etiology

• Human parvovirus B19

Transmission

- Unknown (possible respiratory and blood)

Incubation

- 4 to 14 days

Period of Communicability

- Up to 1 week after onset of symptoms

Manifestations

- Rash appears in three stages:
  - I: Erythema on face (slapped face appearance) for 1 to 4 days
  - II: Maculopapular red spots symmetrically on extremities 1 day after face rash
  - III: Rash subsides (unless irritated by sun or heat)
- Fever, myalgia, lethargy, nausea, and abdominal pain may occur

Interventions

- None required but may use antipyretics or analgesics for comfort

German Measles/Rubella

A mild viral infection that primarily affects the skin and lymph nodes.

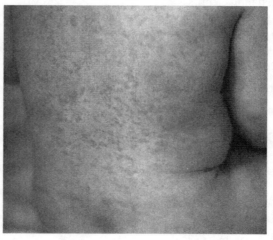

Source: http://upload.wikimedia.org/wikipedia/commons/b/be/Rash_of_rubella_on_skin_of_child%27s_back.JPG

Etiology

- Rubella virus

Transmission

- Direct contact or via articles contaminated with nasopharyngeal secretions, feces, or urine

Incubation

- 14 to 21 days

Period of Communicability

- 7 days before and 5 days after rash

Manifestations

- Low-grade fever, headache, anorexia, conjunctivitis, lymphadenopathy, and cold symptoms lasting 1 to 5 days prior to rash (these symptoms are often absent in children)
- Pinkish red maculopapular rash on the face that spreads rapidly downward. Disappears in the same order; usually gone by third day

FAST FACTS in a NUTSHELL

Pediatric nurses should have titers to ensure immunity to rubella.
Care is taken to avoid exposing the virus to pregnant women, since infection of the mother during the first 20 weeks of pregnancy can be serious, resulting in the child being born with congenital rubella syndrome, or result in spontaneous abortion.

Interventions

- Antipyretics and analgesics for symptoms
- Isolate from pregnant women

Lyme Disease

Lyme disease is a bacterial infection transmitted by a tick that can affect different body systems, such as the nervous system, joints, skin, and heart.

Etiology

- *Borrelia burgdorferi*

Transmission

- From the saliva and feces of ticks, especially deer ticks

Incubation

- 3 to 32 days following bite

Manifestations

- Stage 1: Erythema chronicum migrans (ECM) at site of bite; small red papule that enlarges in circumference to a ring with raised, edematous, doughnut-like border; burning feeling
- Stage 2: Neurological—headache, meningoencephalitis, cranial nerve palsies. Cardiac—syncope, heart block, palpitations, severe bradycardia, chest pain, and dyspnea
- Stage 3: Musculoskeletal pain, chronic arthritis

Interventions

- Children older than 8 years: Treat with doxycycline or amoxicillin at time of rash
- Children less than 8 years: Treat with amoxicillin or penicillin

Measles/Rubeola

Caused by the paramyxovirus and is the most unpleasant and the most dangerous of the children's diseases that result in a rash.

Source: http://en.wikipedia.org/wiki/File:Morbillivirus_measles_infection.jpg

Etiology

- Virus

Transmission

- Direct contact with droplet of infected person

Incubation

- 10 to 20 days

Period of Communicability

- 4 days before to 5 days after rash

Manifestations

- Fever, cough, conjunctivitis, photophobia
- Koplik spots (small white spots) on buccal mucosa
- Erythematous maculopapular rash on face that gradually spreads downward; less intense in later sites. After 3 to 4 days, brownish in appearance with desquamation in areas of extensive involvement
- Anorexia, malaise, and general lymphadenopathy

Interventions

- Antipyretics and symptomatic care

Mumps

An acute contagious viral illness marked by swelling, especially of the parotid glands.

Etiology

- Paramyxovirus

Transmission

- Droplet or direct contact with saliva

Incubation

- 14 to 21 days

Period of Communicability

- Before swelling and until after swelling subsides

Manifestations

- Fever, headache, anorexia then jaw or ear pain aggravated by chewing
- By third day, glands enlarge (unilateral or bilateral)

Interventions

- Analgesics, antipyretics, encourage fluids

Poliomyelitis

A viral illness that can cause mild to paralytic symptoms. Rare with immunization.

Etiology

- Enteroviruses

Transmission

- Direct contact; spread via fecal–oral and pharyngeal–oropharyngeal routes

Incubation

- 7 to 14 days

Period of Communicability

- One week for throat, 4 to 6 weeks for feces

Manifestations

- Fever, headache, abdominal pain
- Stiffness of neck, back, and legs; paralysis

Interventions

- Isolate the child and provide supportive care (no cure)
- Analgesics and bed rest
- Observe for respiratory distress
- Physical therapy for range-of-motion exercises and positioning techniques

Roseola/Exanthema Subitum

A viral infection that begins with a sudden high fever and is followed by the appearance of a rose-colored rash.

Etiology

- Human herpes virus type 6 (HHV-6)

Transmission

- Unknown (occurs between 6 months and 3 years of age)

Incubation

- 5 to 15 days

Period of Communicability

- Unknown

Manifestations

- High fever (103° F to 105° F) then fever drops rapidly when rash appears
- Maculopapular rash, blanches easily, nonpruritic

Interventions

- Antipyretics (high fever may precipitate febrile seizures)

Scarlet Fever

A group A *streptococcus* infection in which the bacteria make a toxin (poison) that can cause a scarlet-colored rash.

Etiology

- Group A beta-hemolytic streptococci

Transmission

- Direct contact with infected person or infected articles, droplet

Incubation

- 2 to 5 days

Period of Communicability

- During incubation and clinical illness

Manifestations

- High fever, vomiting, headache, chills, malaise, abdominal pain
- Tonsils enlarge, covered with patches of exudate
- Pharynx beefy, red, and edematous
- White strawberry tongue Days 4 to 5; white coat sloughs off, leaving red strawberry tongue
- Palate covered with erythematous punctate lesions
- Red pinpoint rash, flushed face, and circumoral pallor with desquamation by end of week

Interventions

- Nose and throat culture for *Streptococcus* and treat with antibiotics

Whooping Cough/Pertussis

A highly contagious respiratory disease known for uncontrollable, violent coughing.

Etiology

- *Bordetella pertussis*

Transmission

- Droplet, direct or indirect contact with infected articles

Incubation

- 5 to 21 days (usually 10 days)

Period of Communicability

- Before onset of paroxysms to fourth week after onset

Manifestations

- Upper respiratory tract infection: coughing, sneezing, low-grade fever for 1 to 2 weeks
- Dry hacking cough, mostly at night, with high-pitched whoop during paroxysms. This stage can last 4 to 6 weeks
- Vomiting often follows attacks

Interventions

- Cool mist tent, hydration, and antimicrobial therapy

Sexually Transmitted Infections (STIs)

STI is a general term given to infections spread through direct sexual activity. Children and adolescents who are sexually active are subject to acquiring STIs. Newborns are susceptible to ophthalmic neonatorum eye infection and human immunodeficiency virus (HIV) caused by contact with an infected mother at birth.

Human Papillomavirus (HPV)/Condylomata Acuminate/Genital Warts

Etiology

- Most common STI in the United States
- HPV viruses (70 types); some types associated with cervical cancer

Incubation

- May take 3 to 6 months after initial contact for genital warts to present

Manifestations

- Some will remain asymptomatic
- Dry, wart-like growths on vagina, labia, cervix, perineum, penis, scrotum, or anus
- Cervical dysplasia and carcinoma

Interventions

- Cryotherapy, electrocautery, laser, or podophyllin
- More frequent Papanicolaou (Pap) tests once identified

Gonorrhea

Etiology

- *Neisseria gonorrhoeae*

Incubation

- Symptoms can develop 1 day up to 2 weeks after contact
- Large numbers of people remain asymptomatic

Manifestations

- Purulent discharge, painful urination, dyspareunia

Interventions

- Antibiotics
- All newborns are given prophylactic antibiotic eye care to prevent ophthalmia neonatorum (caused by gonorrhea and or chlamydia infections passed from the mother to baby during the birthing process)

Herpes Simplex Virus/Herpes Genitalis (HSV)

Etiology

- Herpes virus type I: Cold sore, fever blister
- Herpes virus type II: Genital

Incubation

- Spread by direct contact
- Can be infectious even when no symptoms are present

═══════════════════════════════*FAST FACTS in a NUTSHELL*

The herpes simplex virus lies dormant in nerve cells until it is activated by stress, sun exposure, menstruation, fever, and/or other stressors.

Manifestations

- Clusters of painful vesicles on lips, vulva, perineum, and anal areas
  - Intense burning, itching at site of outbreak
  - First lesions more painful; recurrent lesions resolve more quickly
- Vesicles rupture in 1 to 7 days and heal in 12 days

Interventions

- No cure; acyclovir (Zovirax, Valtrex) reduces symptoms

- Correct and consistent use of latex condoms can reduce the risk of transmission of genital herpes in children/adolescents who are sexually active

Human Immunodeficiency Virus (HIV)

Etiology

- HIV-1 more prevalent in the United States
- HIV-2 more prevalent in Africa

Transmission

- During pregnancy, childbirth, or breastfeeding if mother is infected
  - Babies have contact with amniotic fluid and blood throughout pregnancy
  - Infected breast milk
- Sexual contact with infected person
- Use of contaminated needles or contact with infected blood

Incubation

- Infants infected at birth may become clear of antibodies in about 15 months

FAST FACTS in a NUTSHELL

Children do not get HIV from casual relationships or through contact at school, home, or within the community.

Manifestations

- Initial symptoms in infancy are vague: Failure to thrive, lymphadenopathy, chronic sinusitis, hepatosplenomegaly, chronic diarrhea, and developmental delay
- Opportunistic infections: Oral thrush, *Pneumocystis jiroveci* pneumonia, herpes viruses, and cytomegalovirus
- Serious bacterial infections: Meningitis, impetigo, urinary tract infections are seen in children

Interventions

- Slow the growth of the virus with prescribed antiviral drugs
- Promote normal growth and development through normal activities and play
- Prevent infections through frequent handwashing and avoidance of contact with sick family members/friends
- Provide healthy nutrition with adequate intake of protein and nutrients

CONCLUSION

The nurse needs to possess basic information regarding common communicable disorders in children, the methods of transmission, and precautions in preventing spread during periods of communicability. Education and open communication are key in the prevention of communicable disorders in children.

REFERENCES AND FURTHER READING

Centers for Disease Control and Prevention. (2013). *Index for diseases and conditions.* Retrieved from http://www.cdc.gov/DiseasesConditions

Hockenberry, M., & Wilson, D. (2013). *Wong's essentials of pediatric nursing* (9th ed.). St. Louis, MO: Elsevier.

Leifer, G. (2011). *Introduction to maternity & pediatric nursing* (6th ed.). St. Louis, MO: Elsevier.

Appendices

Standard Precautions and Transmission-Based Isolation Precautions

In addition to consistent use of standard precautions, additional precautions may be warranted in certain situations, as described below.

A. Identifying Potentially Infectious Patients
- Facility staff remain alert for any patient arriving with symptoms of an active infection (e.g., diarrhea, rash, respiratory symptoms, draining wounds, or skin lesions)
- If patient calls ahead:
  - Have patients with symptoms of active infection come at a time when the facility is less crowded, if possible
  - Alert registration staff ahead of time to place the patient in a private examinatoin room upon arrival if available and follow the procedures pertinent to the route of transmission as specified below

B. Contact Precautions
- Attend to patients with any of the following conditions and/or diseases:
  - Presence of stool incontinence (may include patients with norovirus, rotavirus, or *Clostridium difficile*), draining wounds, uncontrolled secretions, pressure ulcers, or presence of ostomy tubes and/or bags draining body fluids
  - Presence of generalized rash or exanthems
- Prioritize placement of patients in an examination room if they have stool incontinence, draining wounds and/or skin lesions that cannot be covered, or uncontrolled secretions

- Perform hand hygiene before touching the patient and prior to wearing gloves
- Personal protective equipment (PPE) use:
  - Wear gloves when touching the patient and the patient's immediate environment or belongings
  - Wear a gown if substantial contact with the patient or his or her environment is anticipated
- Perform hand hygiene after removal of PPE
- Clean/disinfect the examination room
- Instruct patients with known or suspected infectious diarrhea to use a separate bathroom, if available; clean/disinfect the bathroom before it can be used again

C. Droplet Precautions
- Apply to patients known or suspected to be infected with a pathogen that can be transmitted by droplet route; these include, but are not limited to:
  - Respiratory viruses (e.g., influenza, parainfluenza virus, adenovirus, respiratory syncytial virus, or human metapneumovirus)
  - *Bordetella pertusis*
  - For first 24 hours of therapy: *Neisseria meningitides*, group A *Streptococcus*
- Place the patient in an examination room with a closed door as soon as possible (prioritize patients who have excessive cough and sputum production); if an examination room is not available, the patient is provided a face mask and placed in a separate area as far from other patients as possible while awaiting care
- PPE use:
  - Wear a face mask, such as a procedure or surgical mask, for close contact with the patient; the face mask should be donned upon entering the examination room
  - If substantial spraying of respiratory fluids is anticipated, gloves and gown as well as goggles (or face shield in place of goggles) should be worn
- Perform hand hygiene before and after touching the patient and after contact with respiratory secretions and contaminated objects/materials
- Instruct the patient to wear a face mask when exiting the examination room, avoid coming into close contact with other patients, and practice respiratory hygiene and cough etiquette
- Clean and disinfect the examination room

D. Airborne Precautions
- Apply to patients known or suspected to be infected with a pathogen that can be transmitted by airborne route; these include, but are not limited to:
  - Tuberculosis
  - Measles
  - Chickenpox (until lesions are crusted over)
  - Localized (in immunocompromised patient) or disseminated herpes zoster (until lesions are crusted over)
- Have patient enter through a separate entrance to the facility (e.g., dedicated isolation entrance), if available, to avoid the reception and registration area
- Place the patient immediately in an airborne infection isolation room (AIIR)
- If an AIIR is not available:
  - Provide a face mask (e.g., procedure or surgical mask) to the patient and place the patient immediately in an examination room with a closed door
  - Instruct the patient to keep the face mask on while in the exam room, if possible, and to change the mask if it becomes wet
  - Initiate protocol to transfer patient to a health care facility that has the recommended infection-control capacity to properly manage the patient
- PPE use:
  - Wear a fit-tested N-95 or higher-level disposable respirator, if available, when caring for the patient; the respirator should be donned prior to room entry and removed after exiting the room
  - If substantial spraying of respiratory fluids is anticipated, gloves and gown as well as goggles or face shield should be worn
- Perform hand hygiene before and after touching the patient and after contact with respiratory secretions and/or body fluids and contaminated objects/materials
- Instruct the patient to wear a face mask when exiting the exam room, avoid coming into close contact with other patients, and practice respiratory hygiene and cough etiquette
  - Once the patient leaves, the examination room should remain vacant for generally 1 hour before anyone enters; however, adequate wait time may vary depending on the ventilation rate of the room and should be determined accordingly (Curry, n.d.).

- If staff must enter the room during the wait time, they are required to use respiratory protection

REFERENCES AND FURTHER READING

Centers for Disease Control and Prevention. (2014). *Transmission based precautions*. Retrieved from http://www.cdc.gov/HAI/settings/outpatient/basic-infection-control-prevention-plan-2011/transmission-based-precautions.html

Curry, F. J. (n.d.). National Tuberculosis Center, FAQ: "How long does it take to clear the air in an isolation or high-risk procedure room?"

B

Modified Checklist for Autism in Toddlers, Revised

PERMISSIONS FOR USE OF THE M-CHAT-R/F™

The Modified Checklist for Autism in Toddlers, Revised with Follow-Up (M-CHAT-R/F; Robins, Fein, & Barton, 2009) is a 2-stage parent-report screening tool to assess risk for Autism Spectrum Disorder (ASD). The M-CHAT-R/F is available for free download for clinical, research, and educational purposes. Download of the M-CHAT-R/F and related material is authorized from www.mchatscreen.com.

The M-CHAT-R/F is a copyrighted instrument, and use of the M-CHAT-R/F must follow these guidelines:

1. Reprints/reproductions of the M-CHAT-R must include the copyright at the bottom (© 2009 Robins, Fein, & Barton). No modifications can be made to items, instructions, or item order without permission from the authors.

2. The M-CHAT-R must be used in its entirety. Evidence indicates that any subsets of items do not demonstrate adequate psychometric properties.

3. Parties interested in reproducing the M-CHAT-R/F in print (e.g., a book or journal article) or electronically for use by others (e.g., as part of digital medical record or other software packages) must contact Diana Robins to request permission (DianaLRobins@gmail.com).

4. If you are part of a medical practice, and you want to incorporate the first stage M-CHAT-R questions into your own practice's electronic medical record (EMR), you are welcome to do so. However, if you ever want to distribute your EMR page outside of your practice, please contact Diana Robins to request a licensing agreement.

INSTRUCTIONS FOR USE

The M-CHAT-R can be administered and scored as part of a well-child care visit, and also can be used by specialists or other professionals to assess risk for ASD. The primary goal of the M-CHAT-R is to maximize sensitivity, meaning to detect as many cases of ASD as possible. Therefore, there is a high false positive rate, meaning that not all children who score at risk will be diagnosed with ASD. To address this, we have developed the Follow-Up questions (M-CHAT-R/F). Users should be aware that even with the Follow-Up, a significant number of the children who screen positive on the M-CHAT-R will not be diagnosed with ASD; however, these children are at high risk for other developmental disorders or delays, and therefore, evaluation is warranted for any child who screens positive. The M-CHAT-R can be scored in less than two minutes. Scoring instructions can be downloaded from http://www.mchatscreen.com. Associated documents will be available for download as well.

SCORING ALGORITHM

For all items except 2, 5, and 12, the response "NO" indicates ASD risk; for items 2, 5, and 12, "YES" indicates ASD risk. The following algorithm maximizes psychometric properties of the M-CHAT-R:

LOW-RISK: Total Score is 0–2; if child is younger than 24 months, screen again after second birthday. No further action required unless surveillance indicates risk for ASD.

MEDIUM-RISK: Total Score is 3–7; Administer the Follow-Up (second stage of M-CHAT-R/F) to get additional information about at-risk responses. If M-CHAT-R/F score remains at 2 or higher, the child has screened positive. Action required: refer child for diagnostic evaluation and eligibility evaluation for early intervention.

If score on Follow-Up is 0–1, child has screened negative. No further action required unless surveillance indicates risk for ASD. Child should be rescreened at future well-child visits.

HIGH-RISK: Total Score is 8–20; It is acceptable to bypass the Follow-Up and refer immediately for diagnostic evaluation and eligibility evaluation for early intervention.

M-CHAT-R™

Please answer these questions about your child. Keep in mind how your child <u>usually</u> behaves. If you have seen your child do the behavior a few times, but he or she does not usually do it, then please answer **no.** Please circle **yes** or **no** for every question. Thank you very much.

1.	If you point at something across the room, does your child look at it? (FOR EXAMPLE, if you point at a toy or an animal, does your child look at the toy or animal?)	Yes	No
2.	Have you ever wondered if your child might be deaf?	Yes	No
3.	Does your child play pretend or make-believe? (FOR EXAMPLE, pretend to drink from an empty cup, pretend to talk on a phone, or pretend to feed a doll or stuffed animal?)	Yes	No
4.	Does your child like climbing on things? (FOR EXAMPLE, furniture, playground equipment, or stairs)	Yes	No
5.	Does your child make <u>unusual</u> finger movements near his or her eyes? (FOR EXAMPLE, does your child wiggle his or her fingers close to his or her eyes?)	Yes	No
6.	Does your child point with one finger to ask for something or to get help? (FOR EXAMPLE, pointing to a snack or toy that is out of reach)	Yes	No
7.	Does your child point with one finger to show you something interesting? (FOR EXAMPLE, pointing to an airplane in the sky or a big truck in the road)	Yes	No

(continued)

(continued)

8. Is your child interested in other children? (FOR EXAMPLE, does your child watch other children, smile at them, or go to them?)   Yes   No

9. Does your child show you things by bringing them to you or holding them up for you to see—not to get help, but just to share? (FOR EXAMPLE, showing you a flower, a stuffed animal, or a toy truck)   Yes   No

10. Does your child respond when you call his or her name? (FOR EXAMPLE, does he or she look up, talk or babble, or stop what he or she is doing when you call his or her name?)   Yes   No

11. When you smile at your child, does he or she smile back at you?   Yes   No

12. Does your child get upset by everyday noises? (FOR EXAMPLE, does your child scream or cry to noise such as a vacuum cleaner or loud music?)   Yes   No

13. Does your child walk?   Yes   No

14. Does your child look you in the eye when you are talking to him or her, playing with him or her, or dressing him or her?   Yes   No

15. Does your child try to copy what you do? (FOR EXAMPLE, wave bye-bye, clap, or make a funny noise when you do)   Yes   No

16. If you turn your head to look at something, does your child look around to see what you are looking at?   Yes   No

17. Does your child try to get you to watch him or her? (FOR EXAMPLE, does your child look at you for praise, or say "look" or "watch me?"   Yes   No

18. Does your child understand when you tell him or her to do something? (FOR EXAMPLE, if you don't point, can your child understand "put the book on the chair" or "bring me the blanket?"   Yes   No

19. If something new happens, does your child look at your face to see how you feel about it? (FOR EXAMPLE, if he or she hears a strange or funny noise, or sees a new toy, will he or she look at your face?)   Yes   No

20. Does your child like movement activities? (FOR EXAMPLE, being swung or bounced on your knee)   Yes   No

Permissions for Use

The Modified Checklist for Autism in Toddlers, Revised, with Follow-Up (M-CHAT-R/F; Robins, Fein, & Barton, 2009) is designed to accompany the M-CHAT-R. The M-CHAT-R/F may be downloaded from www.mchatscreen.com.

The M-CHAT-R/F is a copyrighted instrument, and use of this instrument is limited by the authors and copyright holders. The M-CHAT-R and M-CHAT-R/F may be used for clinical, research, and educational purposes. Although we are making the tool available free of charge for these uses, this is copyrighted material and it is not open source. Anyone interested in using the M-CHAT-R/F in any commercial or electronic products must contact Diana L. Robins at DianaLRobins@gmail.com to request permission.

Instructions for Use

The M-CHAT-R/F is designed to be used with the M-CHAT-R; the M-CHAT-R is valid for screening toddlers between 16 and 30 months of age, to assess risk for autism spectrum disorder (ASD). Users should be aware that even with the Follow-Up, a significant number of the children who fail the M-CHAT-R will not be diagnosed with ASD; however, these children are at risk for other developmental disorders or delays, and therefore, follow-up is warranted for any child who screens positive.

Once a parent has completed the M-CHAT-R, score the instrument according to the instructions. If the child screens positive, select the Follow-Up items based on which items the child failed on the M-CHAT-R; only those items that were originally failed need to be administered for a complete interview.

Each page of the interview corresponds to one item from the M-CHAT-R. Follow the flowchart format, asking questions until a PASS or FAIL is scored. Please note that parents may report "maybe" in response to questions during the interview. When a parent reports "maybe," ask whether most often the answer is "yes" or "no" and continue the interview according to that response. In places where there is room to report an "other" response, the interviewer must use his/her judgment to determine whether it is a passing response or not.

Score the responses to each item on the M-CHAT-R/F Scoring Sheet (which contains the same items as the M-CHAT-R, but Yes/No has been replaced by Pass/Fail). The interview is considered to be a screen positive if the child fails any two items on the Follow-Up. If a child screens positive on the M-CHAT-R/F, it is strongly recommended that the child is referred for early intervention and diagnostic testing as soon as possible. Please note that if the healthcare provider or parent has concerns about ASDs, children should be referred for evaluation regardless of the score on the M-CHAT-R or M-CHAT-R/F.

M-CHAT-R FOLLOW-UP™ SCORING SHEET

Please note: Yes/No has been replaced with Pass/Fail

1.	If you point at something across the room, does your child look at it? (FOR EXAMPLE, if you point at a toy or an animal, does your child look at the toy or animal?)	Pass	Fail
2.	Have you ever wondered if your child might be deaf?	Pass	Fail
3.	Does your child play pretend or make-believe? (FOR EXAMPLE, pretend to drink from an empty cup, pretend to talk on a phone, or pretend to feed a doll or stuffed animal)	Pass	Fail
4.	Does your child like climbing on things? (FOR EXAMPLE, furniture, playground equipment, or stairs)	Pass	Fail
5.	Does your child make <u>unusual</u> finger movements near his or her eyes? (FOR EXAMPLE, does your child wiggle his or her fingers close to his or her eyes?)	Pass	Fail
6.	Does your child point with one finger to ask for something or to get help? (FOR EXAMPLE, pointing to a snack or toy that is out of reach)	Pass	Fail
7.	Does your child point with one finger to show you something interesting? (FOR EXAMPLE, pointing to an airplane in the sky or a big truck in the road)	Pass	Fail
8.	Is your child interested in other children? (FOR EXAMPLE, does your child watch other children, smile at them, or go to them?)	Pass	Fail

(continued)

9. Does your child show you things by bringing them to you or holding them up for you to see—not to get help, but just to share? (FOR EXAMPLE, showing you a flower, a stuffed animal, or a toy truck)   Pass   Fail

10. Does your child respond when you call his or her name? (FOR EXAMPLE, does he or she look up, talk or babble, or stop what he or she is doing when you call his or her name?)   Pass   Fail

11. When you smile at your child, does he or she smile back at you?   Pass   Fail

12. Does your child get upset by everyday noises? (FOR EXAMPLE, a vacuum cleaner or loud music)   Pass   Fail

13. Does your child walk?   Pass   Fail

14. Does your child look you in the eye when you are talking to him or her, playing with him or her, or dressing him or her?   Pass   Fail

15. Does your child try to copy what you do? (FOR EXAMPLE, wave bye-bye, clap, or make a funny noise when you do)   Pass   Fail

16. If you turn your head to look at something, does your child look around to see what you are looking at?   Pass   Fail

17. Does your child try to get you to watch him or her? (FOR EXAMPLE, does your child look at you for praise, or say "look" or "watch me?")   Pass   Fail

18. Does your child understand when you tell him or her to do something? (FOR EXAMPLE, if you don't point, can your child understand "put the book on the chair" or "bring me the blanket?")   Pass   Fail

19. If something new happens, does your child look at your face to see how you feel about it? (FOR EXAMPLE, if he or she hears a strange or funny noise, or sees a new toy, will he or she look at your face?)   Pass   Fail

20. Does your child like movement activities? (FOR EXAMPLE, being swung or bounced on your knee)   Pass   Fail

Total Score: _____

Index